D0819926

THE
MASTER
PLAN

The Prevention Total Health System®

THE MASTER PLAN

by the Editors of
Prevention® Magazine

Rodale Press, Emmaus, Pennsylvania

Library of Congress Cataloging in Publication Data

The master plan.

(The Prevention total health system)
On t.p. the registered trademark symbol "R" is superscript following "Prevention" in the statement of responsibility and series areas.
Includes index.
1. Health.   2. Medicine, Prevention.   3. Consumer education.   I. Prevention (Emmaus, Pa.)   II. Series.
RA776.M437   1986   613   86-3058
ISBN 0-87857-556-1   hardcover
 4 6 8 10 9 7 5 3   hardcover

NOTICE

The Prevention Total Health System®
Series Editors: William Gottlieb, Mark Bricklin
The Master Plan Editor: Carol Keough
Writers: Mike McGrath (Chapters 1, 7); Sharon Faelten (Chapters 3, 9); Nona Cleland (Chapter 4); G. Ellen Michaud (Chapter 5); Dary Matera (Chapters 6, 8); Patrice Smith (Chapter 10)
Research Chief: Carol Baldwin
Associate Research Chief, Prevention Health Books: Susan Nastasee
Assistant Research Chief, Prevention Health Books: Holly Clemson
Researchers: Jill Jurgensen, Lynda Pollack, Jan Eickmeier, Sally Novack, Ann Gossy
Copy Editor: Jane Sherman
Copy Coordinator: Joann Williams
Series Art Director: Jane C. Knutila
Designers: Lynn Foulk, Alison Lee
Project Assistants: Lisa Gatti, Margot J. Weissman
Illustrators: Bascove, Susan Blubaugh, Mellisa Edmonds, Susan Gray, Lynn Foulk, Mary Anne Shea, Elwood Smith, Wendy Wray
Director of Photography: T. L. Gettings
Photo Editor: Margaret Skrovanek
Staff Photographers: Angelo M. Caggiano, Carl Doney, Donna Hornberger, Alison Miksch
Production Manager: Jacob V. Lichty
Senior Production Coordinator: Barbara A. Herman
Production Coordinator: Eileen F. Bauder
Composite Typesetter: Brenda J. Kline
Production Assistant: Barbara Sellers
Office Personnel: Roberta Mulliner, Janet Schuler

Rodale Books, Inc.
Publisher: Tom Woll
Senior Managing Editor: William H. Hylton
Assistant Managing Editor: Ann Snyder
Art Director: Jerry O'Brien
Director of Marketing: Pat Corpora
Director of Book Production, Trade Sales and Subsidiary Rights: Ellen J. Greene

Rodale Press, Inc.
Chairman of the Board: Robert Rodale
President: Robert Teufel
Executive Vice President: Marshall Ackerman
Group Vice Presidents: Sanford Beldon
                                    Mark Bricklin
Senior Vice President: John Haberern
Vice Presidents: John Griffin
                          James C. McCullagh
                          David Widenmyer
Secretary: Anna Rodale

Contents

Preface

The ABCs and XYZs of Medical Care

The United States has the best legal system in the world. At least that's my opinion. Its teeth grind finer than any other I've seen. Yet it is my devout wish not to get so much as a traffic ticket. I pray I will not be called as a witness. I perform strange and mysterious rites so as not to be audited. I don't want those fine, sharp teeth grinding near *my* bones.

The United States also has the best medical care system in the world. But, save for vaccines and checkups, I want no part of *its* wonders, either. It is my deepest wish that every medical machine that hums and swings on hinges should be seized up by the rust of disuse; that lifesaving drugs should grow moldy in forgotten vials; and that surgeons' deft hands should grow clumsy for lack of patients. Every good doctor should agree; every payer of bills say *amen.* Robert Rodale, the editor of *Prevention,* calls it the prevention of medicine. By that we mean that the ideal we should all aim for is not better medical care but avoiding the need for medical care in the first place.

Ideally, the chief purpose of our wonderful medical care system ought be to keep people out of it. But the overwhelming emphasis winds up on treatment of disease and injury, not their prevention.

Here and there, medical centers are beginning to take prevention seriously, but we have a long way to go. And no wonder. With so much money going for treatment, there seems to be none "left over" to teach health. Yet, the money it takes to treat just one single victim of serious heart disease could be used to personally and intensively educate perhaps 250 people how to avoid circulatory disease. Instead of begging for "leftover money," prevention must obviously be made the first priority.

On a more personal level, it's also important to recognize the big difference between medical care and health care. The first is something doctors do. The second is what *you* do, based on medical guidance. And that's what *The Master Plan* is about. Putting all that good guidance—that you may or may not have received from your physician—into a program. A plan you can use. Goals that inspire you. In *The Master Plan,* which sums up The Prevention Total Health System,® we try to do it all.

We clue you in on some of the simplest things you can do to avoid those humming, tilting, blinking machines. Wear a seat belt. Don't smoke. Keep your weight in line. Get some moderate exercise every day. Eat more vegetables, grains, fruit and fish. Those are the ABCs, but they can keep you from the XYZs of medical care.

We also cover the finer points. Specific foods to avoid, and foods that have what your own system may need more of. The most useful medical tests for people of different ages and situations. New trends that make sense, and trends that make trouble. The unappreciated importance of a happy, tranquil mind, and how you can enjoy both even if you're working harder than ever.

This book is the capstone of perhaps the most complete and practical health resource ever prepared for the public. Read it. Use it. Enjoy it!

Executive Editor, **Prevention**® Magazine

1

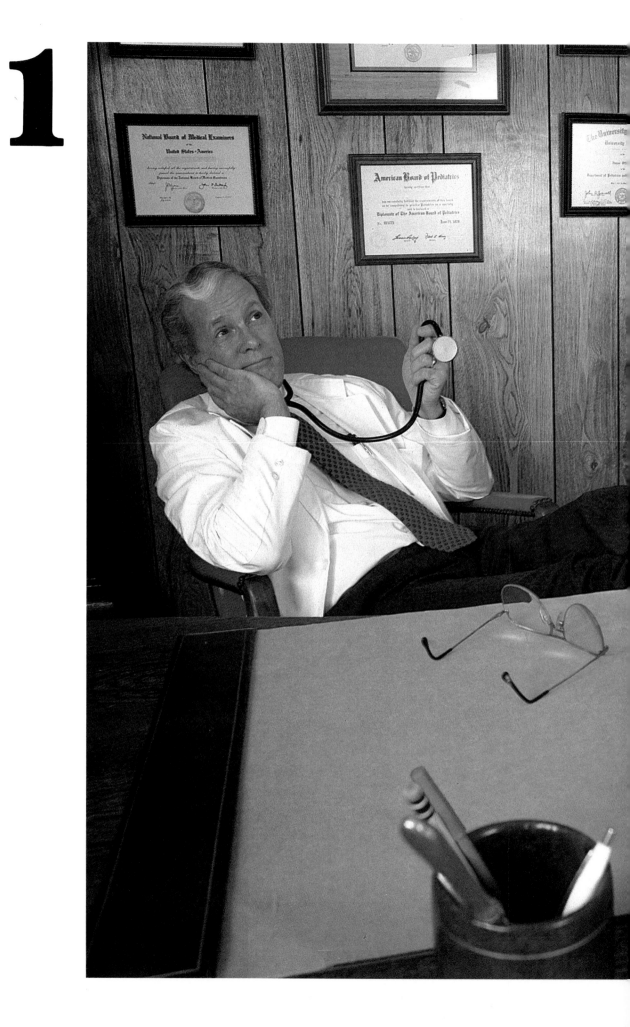

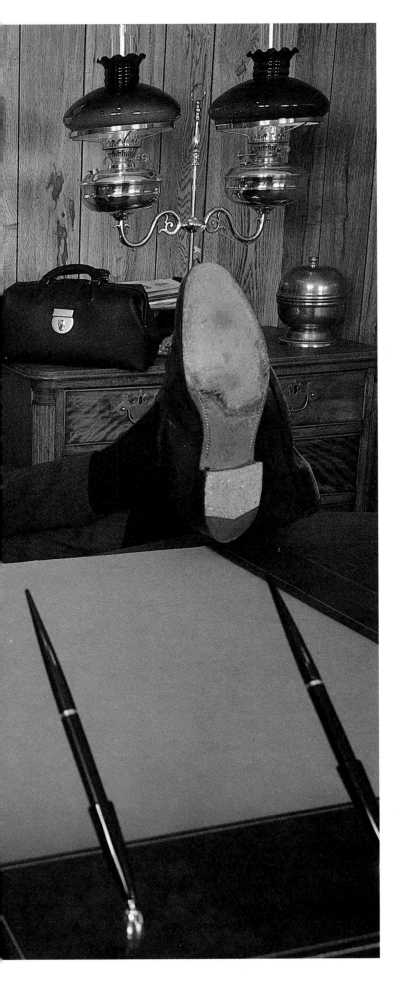

Preventing Medicine

In today's world, the value of an ounce of prevention has become priceless.

Back at the dawn of the age of doctors, Hippocrates had some good advice for the first physicians. "Above all else," he said, "do no harm." He knew that an art created to save lives also had the potential, if used unwisely, to take lives.

Today's doctors sometimes seem oblivious to that simple lesson. People turn to them hoping for an enlightened cure, but they may end up in worse shape than if they had stayed away. It's been estimated that *mistakes* by doctors may be responsible for 5 percent of all hospital admissions.

And it's far from safe once you get inside those hallowed halls of healing, where 20,000 people die needlessly each year from hospital-bred infections. Thousands more are unknowing victims of unnecessary surgery, dangerous tests and improper use of medications.

How do you keep from becoming one of these unfortunate people? Prevention. If they had only taken certain, very specific steps to stay healthy, these people might have avoided the costly and sometimes chancy medical system. The idea is not to avoid doctors, but to avoid *needing* doctors.

Maybe they kept smoking long after they knew they should quit. Maybe they made jokes when they should have made a commitment to exercise. Maybe they forgot to use their seat belts or succumbed to the lure of fudge ripple too often.

If any of these *maybes* sound a little too familiar, consider them to be like short bursts of a warning siren—a call to review and possibly revamp your lifestyle. After all, keeping fit, trim, smoke free and buckled up (along with other prevention-minded habits) are all *sure* ways to protect or improve your health. Certainly an admirable goal in its own right, good health also allows you to have more control over your life (and even more money in your pocket).

That's what we want to help you achieve with this book—better health and a better life. *That's* the Master Plan!

WHO POCKETS YOUR PAYCHECK?

"Billions and *billions*!"

That's not astronomer Carl Sagan guessing the number of stars in the universe. It's Eugene D. Robin, M.D., estimating the amount of money wasted in the U.S. each year on useless tests and unnecessary medical procedures.

"We spend about $350 billion a year on health care," figures Dr. Robin, a professor of medicine and physiology at Stanford University School of Medicine. "Let's be very conservative and say that just 20 percent of that sum is unnecessary. It still amounts to $66 billion a year!"

If Dr. Robin is correct, every man, woman and child in America wastes about $330 a year on unnecessary medical care. This sum does not include the cost of any kind of necessary or even marginally useful medicine. (In fact, seeing a doctor when you need one can prevent more serious problems in the future.) Instead it represents the amount wasted, for example, on surgery performed because the surgeon needs the work or on tests that you have to endure even though the results will make no difference in your treatment.

"If we simply cut out tests that are obviously unnecessary," estimates Dr. Robin, "we could probably save $50 billion a year. I think it's fair to say that the average family would save hundreds of dollars and some not-so-average families might save thousands."

The savings would be most obvious in "out-of-pocket" expenses. That's the money that goes out of your pocket and into someone else's. It may *seem* like medical insurance covers all costs, but most people still pay cash in addition to insurance premiums.

In fact, one out of every ten American families spends *more* than 10 percent of their income on these out-of-pocket expenses, according to the National Center for Health Services, Research and Health Care Technology Assessment. Worse, nearly half of this group spends a whopping 20 percent or more of their income on medical care instead of on vacations or a nicer place to live.

Even if you're not paying extreme amounts in out-of-pocket expenses, you probably have felt the sharp pinch of medical care costs. And that's not surprising. The nation's medical bill rose from about $27 billion in 1960 to $75 billion in 1970 to $247 billion in 1980, a nearly tenfold increase.

And even the expenses that are covered by insurance are hardly free. The huge premiums your employer has to pay leave less money available for employee raises and other benefits. And for most people there are still expenses that are not covered, in addition to copayments and deductibles.

But you've already taken the first step toward saving some of that money—just by reading this book.

The president of the Center for Corporate Health Promotion, Donald Vickery, M.D., estimates that for every dollar you spend on materials to help educate yourself about good

Every year, there are more and more doctors available for each possible patient. Although some critics view this oversupply as a potential problem, it's also a solution for those who aren't happy with their current physician. More doctors, after all, means more choices—for you!

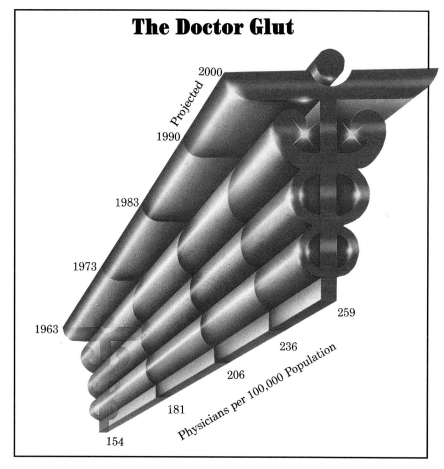

The Doctor Glut

2000
1990 Projected
1983
1973
1963

259
236
206
181
154

Physicians per 100,000 Population

health, you save $3 to $4 in medical costs.

LET THE BUYER BEWARE

Sure, health care is expensive, but money is only a small part of what you pay. Today's medical system may be as hazardous to your health as it is to your wallet.

Take, for example, the problem of infections. These are not problems the hospital failed to cure. These are infections originating in the hospital, infections the patient would never have gotten if he had simply stayed out of the hospital to begin with.

Some people in the health care industry have labeled them nosocomial infections, a convenient name because the general public doesn't know what it means. But an infection by any name can be deadly. In fact, it could well be among the ten leading causes of death in the U.S., according to the *American Journal of Epidemiology.*

It is both surprising and ironic that being a patient in a hospital could expose you to one of the most frequent causes of death in this country. But infections aren't the only problem.

"Accidents that vary from minor to life-taking are extraordinarily common and occur in all hospitals," says Dr. Robin, author of a book on the subject, *Matters of Life and Death: Risks vs. Benefits of Health Care.* He estimates that "one-third of all patients coming into hospitals will have some kind of mishap."

For somewhere between 5 and 10 percent of those people, the mishap will be life-threatening. And one study revealed that for "as many as 1 or 2 percent, the iatrogenic [caused by the treatment] episode is involved in the death of the patient," says Dr. Robin.

Saying that a patient died as a result of an "iatrogenic episode" sure sounds a lot nicer than admitting that they were killed as a direct result of being hospitalized, but that's exactly what it means. Dr. Robin notes that "standard practices"—not mistakes—contribute heavily to the potential dangers of modern medicine.

Overtesting provides a good example. "A huge majority of the

tests done in doctor's offices and hospitals have absolutely no impact whatsoever on the treatment of the patient," he explains.

Why run tests, including some that are extremely dangerous, when the physician isn't going to treat you any differently no matter what the results?

"Doctors run a lot of unnecessary tests to protect themselves against a malpractice suit," explains Dr. Robin.

Patients themselves are also a part of the problem. "They *want* modern medicine," notes Dr. Robin. That means tests. And prescriptions.

"I think the single greatest risk, one that may account for 60 to 70

A Doctor Diagnoses the Medical Establishment

"Medical students leave school overly impressed with the beneficial effects of the skills they have acquired and too little aware of their capacity to do harm," warns Eugene D. Robin, M.D., professor of medicine and physiology at Stanford University School of Medicine. "By restricting your medical encounters to those that are absolutely necessary, you will be avoiding the risks inherent in most diagnostic and therapeutic procedures." What risks? Here are some of them, according to Dr. Robin:

- "Every test has the potential to cause harm. Complications from being tested and treated unnecessarily can cost you your life."
- "Medicine has no organized system for detecting or recording diagnostic errors, although considerable evidence suggests that these occur frequently."
- "There is an oversupply of doctors. As a result, patients are overdoctored and their best interests may be sacrificed for the economic survival of the doctor."
- "There are too many hospital beds, so patients are overhospitalized, where the tendency to overtest and overtreat flourishes and accidents are extraordinarily common. Like packs of cigarettes, hospitals should be labeled 'potentially dangerous to your health.'"

Unlike cigarettes, though, hospitals are not *always* to be avoided. "Conventional medical care does offer the best possibility of helping those who are truly sick," stresses Dr. Robin.

percent of all accidents that occur in hospitals, is in getting the wrong drug or the wrong dose of a drug," says Dr. Robin. He cites the case of a nurse who was supposed to give a patient 0.20 milligrams of a drug—the contents of 1 vial. She gave him 20 vials.

"Hospitals pay surprisingly little attention to either determining the frequency of these accidents or doing something about them," says Dr. Robin, "and in some areas, the statistics are appalling." It's the same with surgery that's not necessary: "Surgeons, after all, are trained to 'do their thing.' Their 'thing' is operating, not deciding that the patient can get by without it," he says.

How can you protect yourself from overmedication, unnecessary surgery, overtesting and infection? Simple, says Dr. Robin. Stay out of the hospital unless you have no alternative.

"Avoiding the medical system can pay big dividends in a patient's health," says Dr. Robin. "But also be sensitive to the dangers of not seeking medical care when it *is* indicated."

SOME HEALTHY QUESTIONS

If the medical system as it exists today is expensive and quite possibly hazardous to your health, what is the best course of action to avoid becoming ensnared in it?

"Just as we change the oil in an automobile because we don't want engine problems, we can avoid a lot of medical encounters with preventive maintenance," explains James O. Mason, M.D., Dr.P.H., director of the Centers for Disease Control (CDC) in Atlanta.

"By looking at groups of people who have a healthy lifestyle and others with less healthy lifestyles, we see immediately—whether we look at cancer, heart disease or a whole range of the problems that plague mankind today—that there are significant positive differences for those with healthy lifestyles."

But the question that's been debated for years is just *which* preventive measures pay off in the kind of

health that keeps you out of the hands of the system.

Robert Rodale, chairman of the board of Rodale Press and editor of *Prevention* magazine, asked 103 health professionals to come up with the answer. They rated various preventive practices for their effectiveness in leading to increased vitality and longevity.

The end result of that study is revealed in the group of questions on the opposite page. They represent 20 of the most important things you can do to protect yourself against accidents and illness.

MANY STEPS TAKEN

To see just how many Americans followed such practices, the firm of Louis Harris and Associates was hired. They conducted a scientific poll to see what people were really doing to protect their health.

"I was very surprised that people were doing so much," said Rodale after the results were in. Out of a possible "score" of 100, it seemed that the American public was doing about 61 percent of all they could to prevent accidents and illness. Rodale says that he "expected the score to be about 18 or 20 percent.

"It illustrates that much prevention is already going on, and also that so much still remains possible," he says. "But what it mainly shows is that, without the level of prevention that *is* going on, we would be in *really* sad shape as a society.

"It's clear now that our entire health-care system really runs on prevention. If everybody smoked, if everybody drank and then drove, if everybody ate the wrong foods, we would not only be inundated with medical costs but our productivity as a nation would be much, much lower."

Several studies bear out the results. One in particular, a magazine survey, revealed that a full 70 percent of American families have made changes in their eating and food-buying habits over the last two years. Many are buying more fresh foods and eating fewer calories, less salt and more fiber.

One study revealed that the death rate for heart disease has

(continued on page 8)

Test Your Level of Personal Prevention

This quiz is designed to find out if you're the type of person who really *tries* to prevent accidents and illness. Answer the questions below and check your *yes* total to see how you score, then see how you compare with other Americans. The quiz is closely based on a poll by Louis Harris and Associates, designed by R. Barker Bausell, Ph.D.

A Questionnaire

	Yes	No
1. Do you *never* smoke cigarettes?	___	___
2. Do you *never* smoke in bed?	___	___
3. Do you *always* wear a seat belt when riding in the front seat of a car?	___	___
4. Do you *never* drive after drinking?	___	___
5. Do you have smoke detectors at home?	___	___
6. Do you socialize with friends, relatives or neighbors at least once a week?	___	___
7. Do you exercise at least 3 times a week?	___	___
8. Do you drink less than 14 drinks a week, and always less than 5 drinks at one sitting?	___	___
9. Do you take steps to avoid accidents at home?	___	___
10. Do you try *a lot* to cut down on fat in your diet?	___	___
11. Do you stay close to your recommended weight?	___	___
12. Do you have your blood pressure checked at least once a year?	___	___
13. Do you take steps to avoid stress?	___	___
14. Do you try *a lot* to eat enough fiber?	___	___
15. Do you try *a lot* to cut down on cholesterol in your diet?	___	___
16. Do you try *a lot* to get enough vitamins and minerals?	___	___
17. Do you have your teeth checked annually?	___	___
18. Do you try *a lot* to cut down on sodium?	___	___
19. Do you try *a lot* to avoid too much sugar?	___	___
20. Do you get 7 or 8 hours of sleep per night?	___	___

Total number of *yes* answers ___

B Compare Yourself with Other Americans

Your Yes Total	Your Grade	Who Scored Lower Than You*
20	A	100%
19	A	99%
18	A	98%
17	A	96%
16	A	91%
15	B	83%
14	B	75%
13	B	64%
12	C	50%
11	C	38%
10	C	27%
9	C	18%
8	D	9%
7	D	5%
6	D	2%
5	F	1%
4-1	F	0%

*Percentage: This is how you compare with the rest of the population. For example, if your *yes* total was 17, it means you're doing more to prevent accidents and illness than 96 percent of those who were surveyed. So you *deserve* an A!

C How Many Share Your Good Habits?

Socialize with friends	91%	Avoid stress	59%
Never smoke in bed	88%	Get plenty of fiber	59%
Check blood pressure yearly	82%	Cut down on fat	55%
Drink in moderation	82%	Cut down on sodium	53%
Avoid accidents at home	72%	Cut down on sugar	51%
Check teeth annually	71%	Cut down on cholesterol	42%
Never smoke	70%	Exercise 3 times a week	34%
Never drink and drive	68%	Stay close to ideal weight	23%
Have smoke detectors	67%	Always wear seat belts	19%
Get enough sleep	64%		
Get enough vitamins/minerals	63%		

Pitfalls

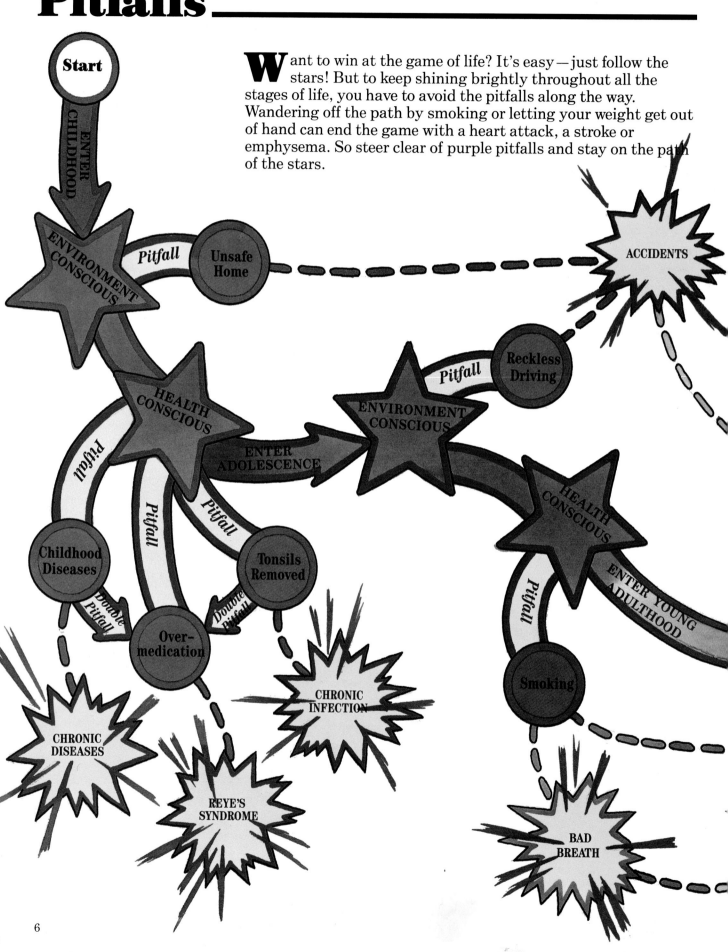

Start

Want to win at the game of life? It's easy—just follow the stars! But to keep shining brightly throughout all the stages of life, you have to avoid the pitfalls along the way. Wandering off the path by smoking or letting your weight get out of hand can end the game with a heart attack, a stroke or emphysema. So steer clear of purple pitfalls and stay on the path of the stars.

ENTER CHILDHOOD

ENVIRONMENT CONSCIOUS

Pitfall — Unsafe Home

ACCIDENTS

HEALTH CONSCIOUS

Pitfall — Reckless Driving

ENVIRONMENT CONSCIOUS

ENTER ADOLESCENCE

Pitfall

Pitfall

Pitfall

HEALTH CONSCIOUS

ENTER YOUNG ADULTHOOD

Childhood Diseases

Tonsils Removed

Double Pitfall

Double Pitfall

Over-medication

Pitfall

Smoking

CHRONIC INFECTION

CHRONIC DISEASES

REYE'S SYNDROME

BAD BREATH

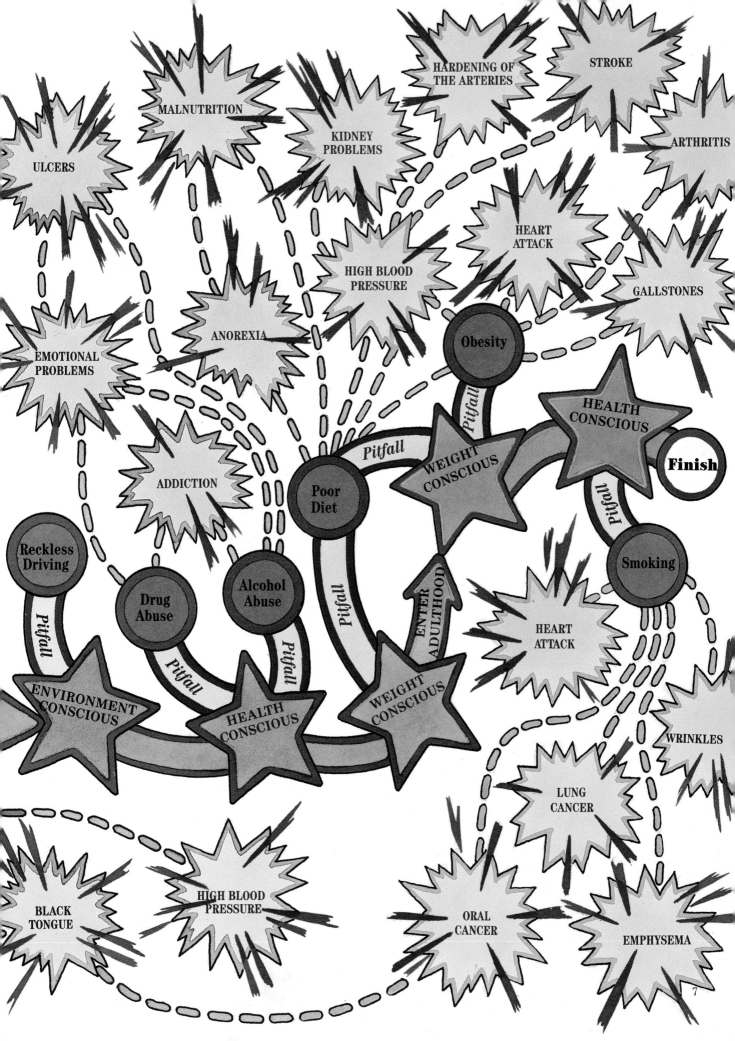

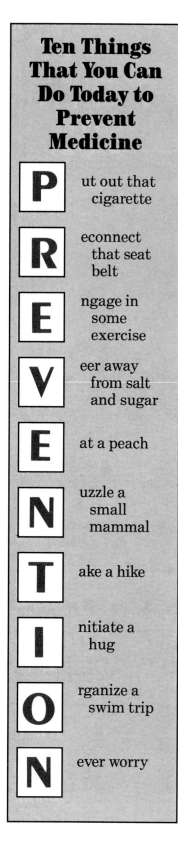

Ten Things That You Can Do Today to Prevent Medicine

P ut out that cigarette

R econnect that seat belt

E ngage in some exercise

V eer away from salt and sugar

E at a peach

N uzzle a small mammal

T ake a hike

I nitiate a hug

O rganize a swim trip

N ever worry

dropped 25 percent and the death rate for strokes has been cut 40 percent since 1970. "These dramatic improvements," says former Health and Human Services Secretary Margaret Heckler, "come in part from Americans' growing interest in taking better care of their own health."

How much better care? According to S. Jay Olshansky, Ph.D., of the University of Utah, the gains we've *already* made have extended our life expectancy as much as if one of the major degenerative diseases had been eliminated from the U.S. In other words, Dr. Olshansky believes that by practicing preventive health care, we can expect to live longer — as much as if someone had discovered a cure for some degenerative diseases, like heart disease or diabetes.

Although we've come a long way in many areas, we're far from perfect in others. One bad habit — smoking — appears to account for projected *increases* in some cancer death rates, particularly those for women.

YOU'VE GONE TOO FAR, BABY

"Lung cancer is about to surpass breast cancer as the leading cause of cancer deaths among women," says Edwin Fisher, Jr., Ph.D., associate professor of psychology and preventive medicine at Washington University in St. Louis. He points out that several surveys show more young women than young men are now taking up the tobacco habit.

"The issue isn't taking risks — that's something that all stimulating and interesting people do," Dr. Fisher insists." The idea is not to take monstrous risks that far outweigh any reward."

With smoking, there appears to be no reward and no end to the risks: lung cancer, obstructive lung disease (chronic bronchitis and emphysema), heart disease and difficulties during pregnancy are all a proven part of the gamble. The final payback, says Dr. Fisher, is that "nonsmokers live five to ten years longer than smokers."

Want to buy back some of that time? It's never too late to stop. Researchers at Yale found that former smokers are no more at risk from heart disease than nonsmokers. Those

who puff away, however, have a 52 percent greater chance of dying from a ticker that just can't take it anymore.

"Even a person who already has chronic lung disease can improve their ability to function and enjoy life," adds Dr. Fisher, who insists that "all other health risks are dwarfed by smoking. There is simply nothing more important that you can do for yourself than to quit."

Some 80 to 90 percent of smokers say that they want to do just that. Dr. Fisher, who chairs the American Lung Association's Smoking or Health Committee, has some tips to help them get what they really crave: freedom.

- Make sure that you want to quit for yourself, and know what your reasons are. They can be for your health, to save money or just to have fresher breath. But you can't quit to please someone else. In fact, spouses shouldn't try to quit together unless both really want to stop.
- Survey your habit. One of the most helpful things you can do is to keep a record for a week of what you're doing and where you are every time you light up. The list that emerges will reveal what things really stimulate your desire to smoke.
- Set a specific date for quitting. It shouldn't be today or tomorrow, since *preparing* to quit is half the battle. Instead, give yourself two to three weeks to get ready.
- Anticipate the temptations and cravings that your list has revealed. Avoid them. If your strongest urge to smoke coincides with after-dinner coffee, for instance, you may have to give up the java for awhile.
- Recruit the support of those around you. Don't be bashful — it's the quitter's right to expect other people to help.
- Be kind to yourself. Since this *is* difficult and one of the most important things you'll ever do, treat it that way. Give yourself presents, treats and favors and don't expect perfection from yourself in other areas. Don't be a hero.
- Don't think that you can quit

without changing parts of your life, at least temporarily. You may have to avoid socializing with friends who still smoke, since they are often the major cause of relapses.

- A relapse *isn't* a failure, so don't panic. Many successful quitters usually have relapsed two or three times before finally succeeding. Learn what beat you this time and work doubly hard to avoid it. Set a new date and start again.
- Never forget that this is a *positive* thing that you're doing. You're not "giving up" anything.

YOUR MOM WAS RIGHT

The years you can add by giving up smoking are just the beginning of the extra time you can buy for yourself, say studies from UCLA and the Human Population Laboratory, California State Department of Health. They kept track of nearly 7,000 people over a period of years and concluded that an average person probably could add *years* to their life by following the simple health practices we learn at our mother's knee.

Specifically, they found that a 45-year-old man who never smoked, maintained his proper weight, ate prudently, slept well, exercised regularly and drank moderately (at most) could expect to live 11 years longer than his counterpart who followed few—or none—of these sound practices.

It's common knowledge, really. More than 90 percent of those polled in a Louis Harris survey agreed with the statement: "If we Americans lived healthier lives, ate more nutritious food, smoked less, maintained our proper weight and exercised regularly, it would do more to improve our health than anything doctors and medicine could do for us."

Take diet, for instance. What you eat, how much you eat and how much you work off can decide to a large degree whether you spend your time being the envy of others or a fixture in the doctor's waiting room.

Want to avoid having to be treated for gallstones? Research published in the *British Medical Journal* suggests you can probably do that just by keeping your weight down, eating less meat, eating more fiber and limiting cholesterol, sugar, saturated fats and alcohol.

Even people who already have arthritis can control its symptoms with a regular program of exercise and weight control. The alternative is to risk the side effects of drugs, gold injections or scarring surgery.

Depressed? Your doctor can put you on drugs or you can spend a lot of money and time on professional counseling—or you can work out. Studies show that aerobic exercise can be a great way to make depressed people feel better.

It's also a good way to lose excess weight, which in turn reduces your chances of encountering a huge variety of medical problems.

Follow the example of 64 patients who had been recommended for heart bypass surgery but instead decided to enter the Pritikin Longevity Center. The low-fat, high-complex-carbohydrate, high-fiber diet, combined with twice-a-day brisk walks, lowered their weight, blood pressure and triglyceride and cholesterol levels within a month.

After five years, those who continued the program's guidelines at home not only had survived without surgery but also saw their health nearly approach that of the general population.

If you're a woman, walking, along with calcium and vitamin D, will also help keep you free of the medical system. How? Because exercise and the right nutrients can help prevent the tragedy of osteoporosis, which weakens bones after menopause.

Understanding the vitamins and minerals that your body needs to stay healthy—and making sure that you get them from food or supplements—can help you avoid a lot of pain and misery in your life. In the case of osteoporosis, for example, proper diet might help prevent a million broken bones and 50,000 premature deaths linked to complications of osteoporosis every year.

The more you know, the more health problems you can avoid. Checking your own blood pressure, for instance, not only keeps you out of the doctor's office directly but can

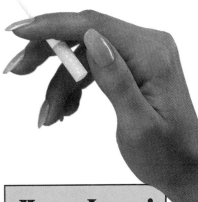

Hocus-Locus!

That craving for a cigarette originates in an area of your brain called the locus ceruleus. Quite coincidentally, a study of 15 people found that a drug used to control high blood pressure, clonidine, may calm it down. The study showed it significantly decreased that craving. However, this is not a cure for smoking. The study warned that smokers will still have to have a lot of personal motivation to quit.

Age and Injury

The charts below show the percentage of deaths in various age groups that result from injuries. Note how injury causes *most* deaths in the young adult years and least in the senior years.

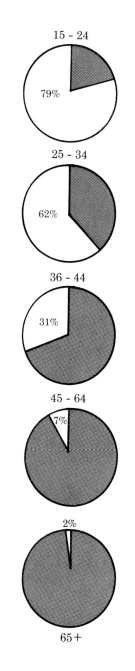

15 - 24

79%

25 - 34

62%

36 - 44

31%

45 - 64

7%

65+

2%

keep you out of the hospital later when you promptly respond to a high reading by reducing both fat and stress in your life. A lack of awareness can result not only in continued high blood pressure but also in a heart attack or stroke.

SAFETY IS NO ACCIDENT

It's even easier to avoid the pain and expense that follows an accident, the fourth leading cause of death in America. All you have to do is pay a little bit of attention and you can avoid the second leading cause of having to see a doctor. What better way to stay out of the medical system?

Accidents and the injuries that result claim more than 94,000 lives a year. They eat up almost 97 billion of our dollars. They account for almost half of all deaths from age 1 to 14, and 51 percent of all deaths from age 15 to 24.

"I'm sure that 50 to 75 percent of the deaths and permanent disability that are injury related could be prevented by the use of simple environmental controls," says Dr. Mason.

He's talking about installing smoke detectors so that you don't sleep through a fire and guardrails to keep you from falling down the stairs or in the tub, tacking down a loose rug so that you don't fall down and go boom, and using your seat belt when you drive.

Seat belts, for example, are remarkably effective. Imagine two separate drivers in the same kind of accident.

According to a government report, the driver who wasn't wearing his belt is pulled from the wreck with fractured vertebrae, multiple cuts and bruises and severe neck strain. He's out of work for a month.

The one who *was* wearing his belt walks away with a couple of bruises. He takes a day off because he's all shook up about what *could* have happened.

Another example, cited by the U.S. Department of Transportation, is a left-front collision, like the one that Barbara Mandrell and her family survived (see "Barbara Mandrell: Saved by a Seat Belt"), except at

much slower speeds.

The person not wearing the seat belt suffers shattered legs and ribs, is out of work for a painful six months and can rack up a total of $43,000 in medical expenses and other costs.

The driver wearing the belt gets out of the car with a stiff neck from a little whiplash instead of being carried off on a stretcher. He misses no time at work.

If the benefits are so great, why do 15,000 people die each year who would survive if they used seat belts? Why do more than a million allow themselves to be more seriously injured than they would be if they buckled up?

"They don't perceive the risks and think that they can get by without using seat belts," answers Dr. Mason. "They just don't realize that they can't control whether or not they have an accident." Even if you were the best driver in the world, he points out, you couldn't do a thing to avoid the drunk who suddenly crosses the center line to come slamming head-on into you.

Even worse, says Dr. Mason, are the mothers who hold small children on their laps instead of strapping them into a safety seat. "They just don't realize the tremendous 'G' forces involved," he explains. "There's no way that they can prevent *themselves* from going forward into the windshield, much less stop their baby from being injured. In fact, it will be *their* body that crushes the child into the windshield as they're thrown forward."

Very few people "refuse" to protect themselves, says the Department of Transportation. They just don't believe that an accident will happen to them. If they believed they were at risk, they'd buckle up. So tape these statistics to the dashboard:

- The impact of hitting the windshield while driving at 30 miles per hour is the same as jumping head-first off a three-story building.
- Most accidents occur close to home and most serious injuries and deaths occur at or under 40 miles per hour.
- The odds say you'll be involved in a crash once every five years.

Wearing a seat belt is the *law* in

Nottingham, England. And since it was enacted, deaths are down an amazing 80 percent. So are neck injuries.

In this country, many companies and communities are offering incentives to drivers who buckle up. They're usually nothing major—free burgers, movie tickets, that kind of thing—but one Pennsylvania hospital, for instance, got more than 90 percent of its employees to buckle up. They may have saved a fortune, since every time an employee dies in a car crash, it costs their company more than $100,000 in medical and other costs.

Of course, a major reason for car accidents is driving after drinking. *Walking* after drinking can also be a problem, observes Dr. Mason.

"The accidents related to alcohol abuse are staggering," he says. "Most people simply don't realize that as few as two drinks can impair their driving skills, or even their ability to negotiate a flight of steps." Another equally serious effect of drinking is that alcohol clouds judgment. "When a person's central nervous system is dulled or depressed by alcohol, you don't get very wise behavior," notes Dr. Mason.

THE MASTER PLAN REVEALED

Promote health. Prevent illness. To do so, must you give up everything you enjoy just to buy a few extra years of monklike misery? Not on your life—which, by the way, we want you to enjoy more than you ever thought possible.

"Once people find the energy to try a different lifestyle, you rarely find them going back to the way they were before," notes Dr. Mason. "You'll often hear them say, 'I wasn't really living then—while I was smoking, food didn't taste as good, I couldn't walk fast without coughing . . .'

"It's the same with every one of the factors we've been talking about," he continues. "People find that they're not giving up *anything*—they're discovering something new and exhilarating that makes the quality of their lives that much better."

And that's the goal of the Master Plan. *Your* goal.

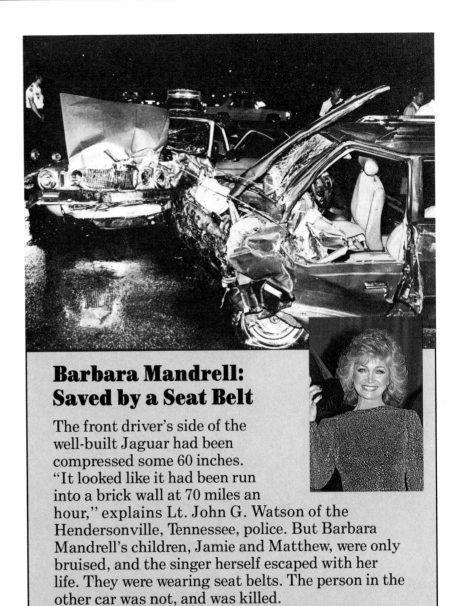

Barbara Mandrell: Saved by a Seat Belt

The front driver's side of the well-built Jaguar had been compressed some 60 inches. "It looked like it had been run into a brick wall at 70 miles an hour," explains Lt. John G. Watson of the Hendersonville, Tennessee, police. But Barbara Mandrell's children, Jamie and Matthew, were only bruised, and the singer herself escaped with her life. They were wearing seat belts. The person in the other car was not, and was killed.

The family usually didn't "buckle up." However, they had been following a station wagon with an open tailgate and watching two children roll around in the back. The sight so unnerved Ms. Mandrell that she turned to the kids and said, "Let's put our seat belts on so *we'll* be safe." Five minutes later a car crossed a center turn lane and hit them head-on. Now, even Barbara's previously unbuckled father wears his seat belt, "which shows that you *can* teach an old dog a new trick," he says.

2

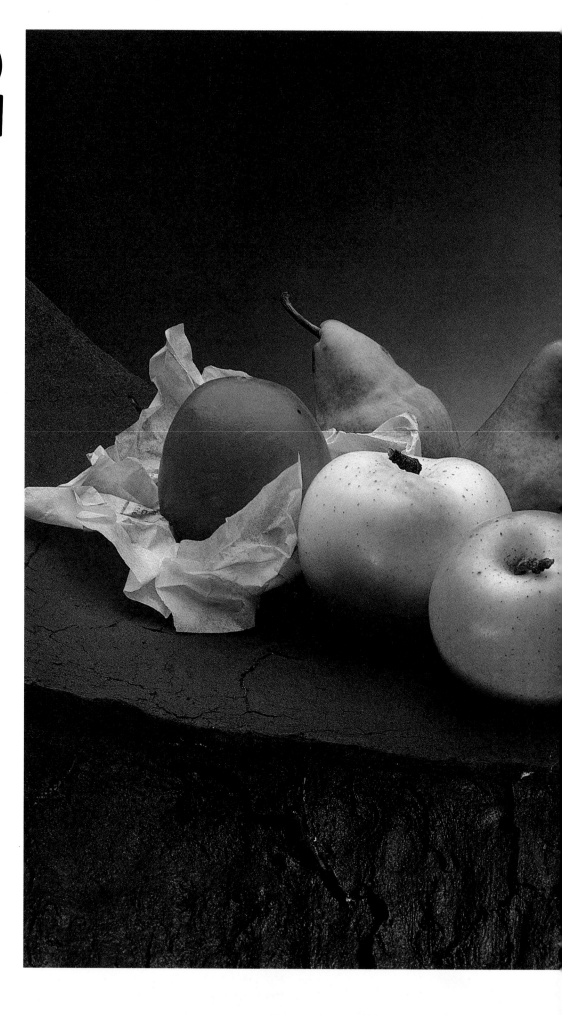

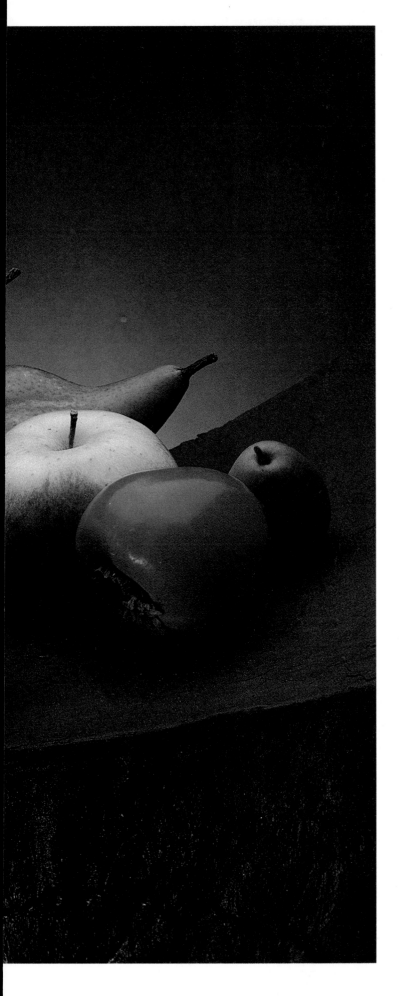

The Nutrition Master Plan

New discoveries in nutritional science help you choose the best foods for total health.

T his breakfast cereal may help prevent cancer, says the TV commercial.

Almost every soft drink on the market is touted for what it *doesn't* contain: no sugar (so it won't rot your teeth), no caffeine (so it won't addle your nerves) and no salt (so it won't mess with your blood pressure).

The word *lite* is used so often it's practically in *Webster's Dictionary.*

Food and health. There's clearly a connection— it's just the *specifics* that aren't so clear. Too much fat is bad—but some kinds of fat are good? Protein is essential—but don't eat too much red meat? Simple carbohydrates, complex carbohydrates— it's enough to give you a complex that you're nutritionally simple-minded.

Well, understanding the food/health connection is really as easy as pie—or at least as easy as four *types* of food, namely the four food groups: meat, dairy, fruits and vegetables, and grains.

We've taken this handy concept—and refurbished it 1980s-style with the latest discoveries in nutritional science. The result is a quick but comprehensive guide to the health values, or lack of them, in every kind of food— your nutritional Master Plan.

MEAT: A CUT ABOVE AVERAGE

Fearful of cholesterol and fat, we've become wary of eating red meat. And make no mistake—you *can* eat too much meat. But if you choose the right cuts, prepare them properly and eat meat in moderation, it can be a positively health-building food. Certain cuts of beef, such as round steak, are fairly lean to begin with, and trimming the fat can reduce them still further. Trim that fat *before* cooking, then broil the steak on a slatted pan so that some of the remaining fat can drain away. The result is good, lean, nutritious eating. (Beef is an extremely good source of protein, B vitamins, iron and zinc.)

However you cut it—or cook it—beef does have more fat than many other foods. But that's true of most protein-rich foods, including dairy products, nuts and seeds. The food that doesn't seem to marry protein and fat is fish. It generally has less fat than meat and is an excellent source of protein. Happily, fish has even more advantages. Would you believe you can help lower your blood pressure and cholesterol and triglyceride levels by eating mackerel and salmon? Researchers worldwide have discovered that certain types of fish—those containing EPA (eicosa-pentaenoic acid, a fatty acid)—may protect against heart disease. Apparently, EPA is a special kind of fat, which researchers at the Oregon Health Sciences University say may be "metabolically unique" and useful in controlling other fats that can clog the bloodstream. Among the fishes favored are mackerel, salmon, bluefish, sardines, herring and tuna. Shellfish, too, are quite low in fat, but the fat they do contain is relatively high in EPA.

DAIRY

News linking calcium deficiency and osteoporosis is no longer buried in medical journals. Today, ads for the mineral even show up on TV. And while calcium supplements certainly ensure that you're getting enough to protect your bones, you still need the vitamin D in milk, which protects against another bone-thinning condition, osteomalacia. Both calcium and vitamin D in milk may also cut the risk of developing colorectal cancer, according to a 20-year study (although the researchers aren't yet sure why).

FRUITS AND VEGETABLES

Ever since we were tykes, we've been told to eat our vegetables. Yet Mom and Dad didn't know then what we know now: Fruits and vegetables may play an important role in warding off cancer. Only recently have scientists discovered that beta-carotene (converted into vitamin A in our bodies), vitamin C and fiber—all found abundantly in various fruits and vegetables—may play special roles in cancer protection.

What *is* it in simple vegetables that could possibly protect against cancer? Beta-carotene, for one thing. One researcher describes it as a shock absorber, protecting the valuable genetic blueprints inside each cell from outside damage.

And vitamin C for another. Found in citrus fruits and melons, as well as vegetables such as broccoli and cabbage, it is a potent antioxidant that may help protect the body against various types of cancer.

GRAINS

Time was, you had to go to a health food store to find foods like brown rice or oat bran. Now supermarkets sell both—and give over their shelves to whole grain cereals, flours and breads. Why the shift?

The simple answer is, "complex." Complex carbohydrates, that is. Like fruits, vegetables and beans, whole grain foods contain fiber, which can lower cholesterol. Oat bran, for example, has been found to lower cholesterol by as much as 13 percent. Increasing your intake of whole grain cereals also will provide a wide range of nutrients, including B vitamins and selenium (which seems to stimulate immunity). Furthermore, by upping the amount of whole grain cereals, breads and pasta you eat, you will be lowering the number of foods in your diet that have a much higher fat content.

SOME HEALTH MYTHS

If you are eating a truly good diet—low in fat, high in complex carbohydrates—will an occasional "recreational" food really do you in? Is a chocolate chip cookie or a glass of beer so terribly unhealthy that it

Various parts of your body rely on specific nutrients to function properly. If you—like the astronauts—want "all systems go," be sure to include foods high in the vitamins and minerals mentioned in the chart on the opposite page as a regular part of your diet.

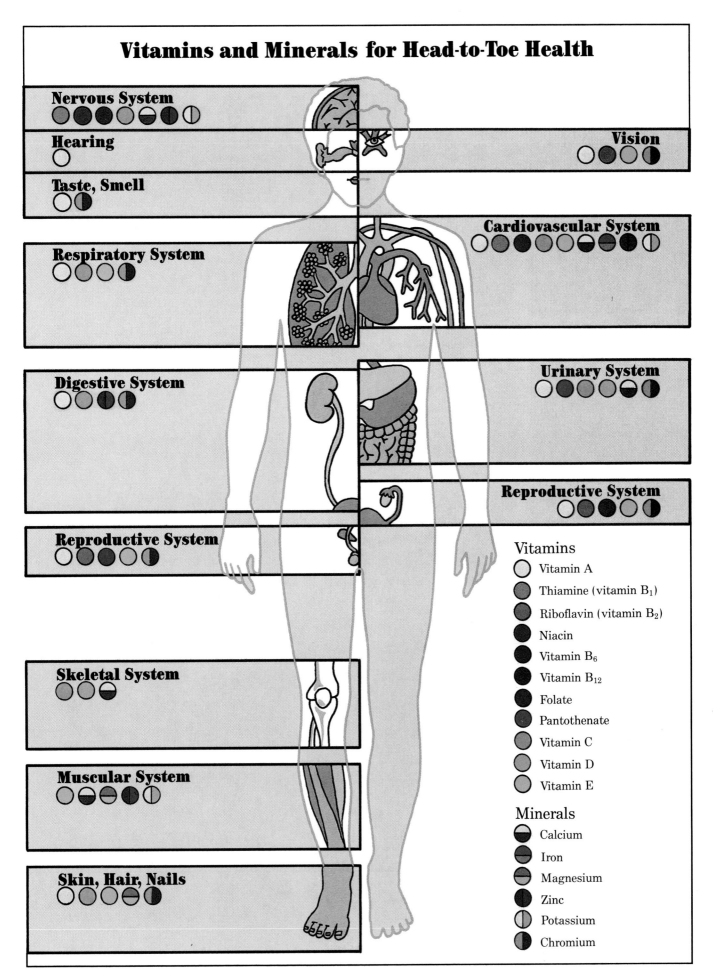

Vitamins and Minerals for Head-to-Toe Health

Nervous System

Hearing

Vision

Taste, Smell

Cardiovascular System

Respiratory System

Digestive System

Urinary System

Reproductive System

Reproductive System

Skeletal System

Muscular System

Skin, Hair, Nails

Vitamins
- Vitamin A
- Thiamine (vitamin B₁)
- Riboflavin (vitamin B₂)
- Niacin
- Vitamin B₆
- Vitamin B₁₂
- Folate
- Pantothenate
- Vitamin C
- Vitamin D
- Vitamin E

Minerals
- Calcium
- Iron
- Magnesium
- Zinc
- Potassium
- Chromium

Can vitamins and minerals help prevent cancer? Apparently so, claims Charles B. Simone, M.D., a cancer specialist. They work in various ways. Some are antioxidants; that is, they can neutralize certain cellular by-products associated with cancer development. Some nutrients actually clear up conditions that threaten to become cancerous, while others suppress "oncogenes," which are thought to cause cancer. Still others work to prevent cancers by strengthening the immune system or working against a virus itself. Finally, one mineral works to cancel out the danger from some toxic metals or chemicals.

cancels all the benefits of the wholesome foods you eat? Let's take an objective look at three favorite health taboos.

Sugar. It rushes into your bloodstream, picks you up and slam-dunks you into the sugar blues. Or so we thought. Newer research, however, reveals that responses to sugar and other carbohydrates vary widely from one person to another. Not everyone reacts to sugar as though it were an amphetamine. Eating candy and other sweets does not condemn you to poor health, as long as you eat them sparingly.

Salt. Sodium—one of the elements in salt—doesn't appear to *cause* high blood pressure. But sodium can *aggra-*

vate the condition in some people, increasing their risk of a stroke. Many people who eat a lot of salt never get high blood pressure. Evidently, much depends on whether or not you are "salt-sensitive," and it may be that only about 10 percent of our population is salt-sensitive.

Alcohol. While overindulgence in alcohol has been linked with high blood pressure and cancers of the esophagus and stomach, light to moderate drinking may not be all that bad. Preliminary research suggests that *low* amounts of alcohol might "relax" some blood vessels, possibly lowering the risk of heart disease and stroke. Some investigators define light to moderate alcohol intake as two or fewer drinks a day.

Nutrients That Protect against Cancer*

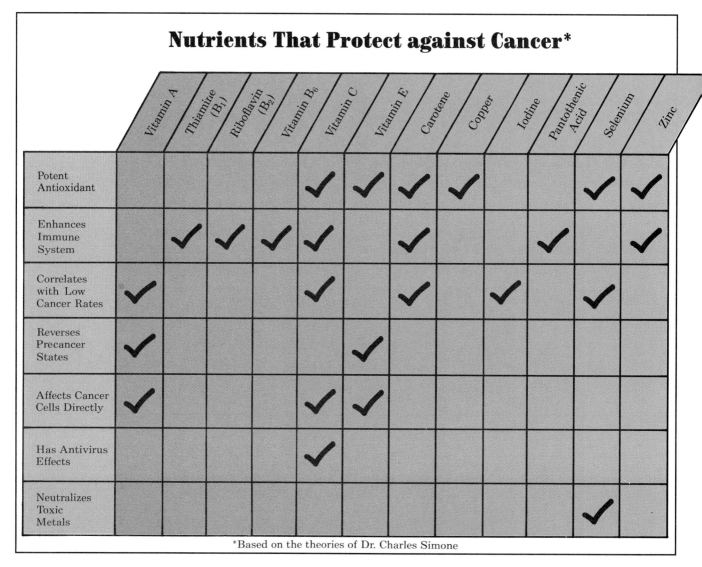

	Vitamin A	Thiamine (B₁)	Riboflavin (B₂)	Vitamin B₆	Vitamin C	Vitamin E	Carotene	Copper	Iodine	Pantothenic Acid	Selenium	Zinc
Potent Antioxidant				✓	✓	✓	✓				✓	✓
Enhances Immune System		✓	✓	✓		✓				✓		✓
Correlates with Low Cancer Rates	✓			✓		✓		✓			✓	
Reverses Precancer States	✓					✓						
Affects Cancer Cells Directly	✓				✓	✓						
Has Antivirus Effects					✓							
Neutralizes Toxic Metals											✓	

*Based on the theories of Dr. Charles Simone

Erin Go Broccoli!

Forget the luck of the Irish—unless there's healthy food cooking in the pot at the end of the rainbow.

A 20-year study of 3 groups of Irish men showed that the men who ate a diet high in saturated fat were 60 percent more likely to die of heart disease than men who didn't. On the other hand, those who ate a diet rich in vegetables and fiber decreased their risk of heart disease by as much as 43 percent.

Each group was judged "high," "medium" and "low" to evaluate their consumption of fat, fiber and vegetables. The charts reveal how these levels affect their risk of heart attack.

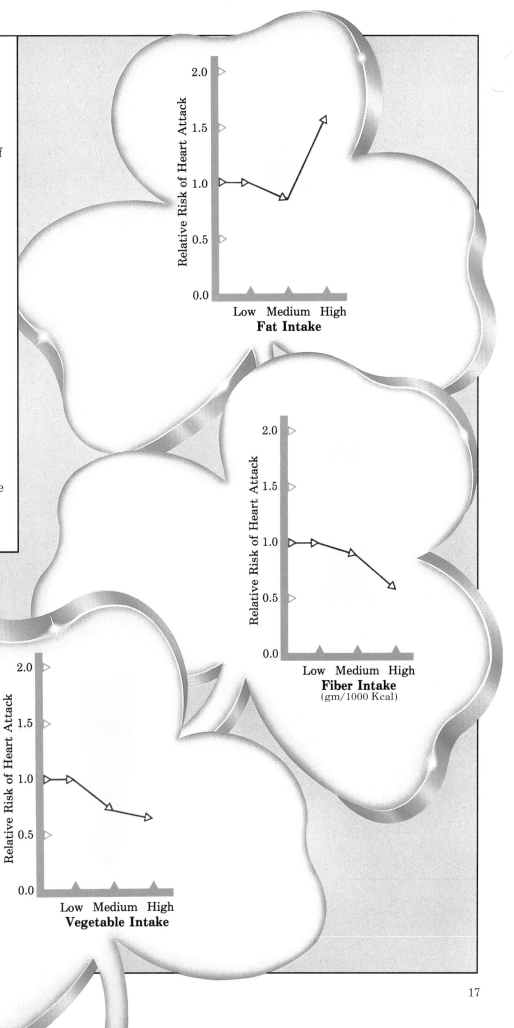

Fat Intake

Fiber Intake
(gm/1000 Kcal)

Vegetable Intake

17

Mastering Weight Control

It's a simple equation: to lose weight, eat less. But that doesn't have to mean eating a less nutritious diet. Just remember to include foods that supply certain specific nutrients. Physicians have found that slight but long-term deficiencies of these key nutrients may lead to certain health or behavior problems, which is just what you don't need when you're trying to diet. Each food listed in the table below contains high levels of at least two of these nutrients.

Take off all your clothes and stand in front of a full-length mirror. Do you like what you see? Or could you stand to lose a few pounds? Or maybe *more* than a few?

If you're overweight, you have company. Studies show that eight out of ten men over 40 years old are overweight. So are seven out of ten women. Not that people aren't concerned about their weight. Quite the contrary: One study found 88 percent of people who were overweight worried about it.

As you might expect, people who aren't overweight tend to live longer than those who are. And they usually have more fun, because they get around more easily, don't have as many aches and pains and worry less—in general, they feel better about themselves. So if you're overweight, you probably want to reduce. If you're not, you'll want to stay that way.

SIZING YOURSELF UP

Where should you stand, weight-wise?

Right in front of that mirror, because your own reflection is the best indicator of whether or not you need to lose weight. A study conducted by Robert H. Brook, M.D., Sc.D., of the UCLA School of Medicine and Public Health, and Anita L. Stewart, Ph.D., of the Rand Corporation, found that most people who are overweight are pretty good judges of their own weight. Those who are truly overweight don't need a diagram or statistics to tell them so— just a mirror.

What should you do if your reflection tells you to lose weight?

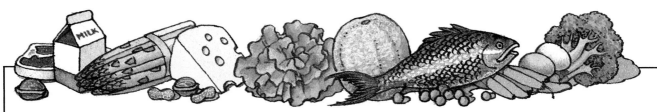

Food Sources of Key Nutrients

	Thiamine (B₁)	Riboflavin (B₂)	B₁₂	Folate	C	Zinc
Asparagus		✗		✗	✗	
Brewer's yeast	✗	✗		✗		
Brussels sprouts				✗	✗	
Cabbage, raw				✗	✗	
Cantaloupe				✗	✗	
Chicken, white meat	✗	✗	✗	✗		✗
Liver, beef	✗	✗	✗	✗		✗
Milk, low fat, 1%	✗	✗	✗			
Orange	✗				✗	
Peppers, green, raw				✗	✗	
Salmon steak	✗	✗	✗			
Soybeans, dried, cooked	✗	✗		✗		✗
Spinach, raw				✗	✗	
Wheat germ, toasted	✗	✗		✗		

Don't Starve Yourself. Cutting back drastically is absolutely the worst way to try to reduce.

The best approach to safe, successful, *permanent* weight control is to learn the caloric and nutritional value of foods and then make intelligent food choices you can stick with for the long haul.

Other helpful tips from weight-loss experts:

Walk a Mile for a Doughnut—Then Skip the Doughnut. There are no two ways about it: Excess calories put on pounds, exercise takes them off. Where to walk and for how long? That's easy: Walk for 30 minutes—away from your house. Somehow, finding the motivation to walk the second 30 minutes (back home) is easy. Do this once a day and you'll lose up to 30 or 40 pounds in a year—without dieting.

Outsmart Restaurant Menus. Ask for simply cooked food. Ask for sauce on the side, not slathered on by the chef (so you can control the amount). Order salads with dressing on the side. Look for fresh fruit desserts. If you like fish, order it often. If you don't like fish, try to learn to like it. Overall, the best cuisines are Chinese or Japanese. The fattiest are Eastern European, Hungarian, German, very posh French food and some kinds of English food. Don't worry about annoying the server—he or she is probably on a diet, too.

Ride Out the Plateaus. All dieters experience weeks where they don't lose an ounce, no matter how carefully they plan their menus or how much they exercise. Don't blow it! Stick with your program and the weight will eventually begin to disappear again.

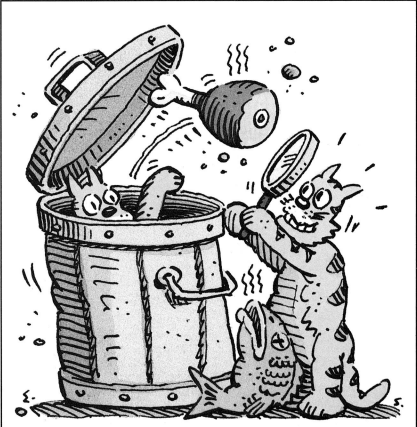

Trashing the Fat

What people throw away can reveal a lot about their health habits. Take meat, for example. People are trimming off an average of 17 percent or more of the separable fat from steaks, chops and other cuts of meat, compared to 3 percent in 1978. So concludes William Rathje, Ph.D., head of a research team that picked through random samples of household trash collected in two western U.S. cities. Evidently, people *are*—quite literally—cutting out fat from their diets.

THIS WAY TO THE MAINTENANCE DEPARTMENT

If the scale still won't budge, get out a measuring tape. Measure your hips. Or your waist. Exercise replaces fat with muscle (which takes up less space), so you could reduce in size without losing pounds.

If the pounds you've lost begin to creep back, you're eating too much or exercising too little—or both. Weigh yourself once a week so things don't get out of hand.

The Master Target

Experts agree that there's no one food that makes or breaks your health and that it's your total diet that keeps you on target. Certainly, emphasize the low-fat, high-fiber, high-nutrient foods in the red circle. But you can also enjoy treats such as cheese, nuts and even porterhouse steak. (For a detailed breakdown, see the list below.)

Eat Frequently

Dairy foods
Low-fat yogurt (plain)
Skim milk

Meat, fish, poultry, eggs
Swordfish*
Salmon*
Trout*
Halibut*
Shrimp*
Chicken (skinned)
Turkey (skinned)
*Broiled, poached, steamed or baked

Vegetables
Red peppers
Kale
Spinach
Broccoli
Acorn squash
Lima beans
Carrots
Brussels sprouts
Navy beans
Cauliflower
Garlic

Fruits
Apricots (dried)
Blackberries
Raspberries
Strawberries
Cantaloupes
Bananas

Grains, breads, cereals
Bran
Amaranth
Millet

Eat Occasionally

Dairy foods
Swiss cheese
Mozzarella (part skim)
Gruyere cheese
Gouda cheese
American cheese

Meat, fish, poultry, eggs
Chicken (with skin)
Turkey (with skin)
Round steak
Chuck roast
Porterhouse steak
Flank steak
Lean ground beef
Leg of lamb
Rump roast (choice)
Veal cutlet
Veal loin
Ham
Pork chops
Pork roast

Grains, breads, cereals
Crackers
Pretzels

Nuts, seeds
Sunflower seeds
Almonds
Pumpkin seeds
Sesame seeds
Peanuts (raw or roasted)
Cashews
Peanut butter

Eat Seldom

Dairy foods
Ice cream
Sherbet

Meat, fish, poultry, eggs
Sturgeon (smoked)
Anchovies
Fish sticks
Duck
Poultry (fried)
Liver
Sirloin steak
Club steak
Lamb ribs
Bologna
Salami
Bacon
Hash
Sausage
Eggs (fried)
Fish (fried)

Vegetables
Vegetables in cream sauce
Fried vegetables

Fruits
Fruit packed in heavy syrup
Fruit drinks
Fruit leather

Grains, breads, cereals
Cookies

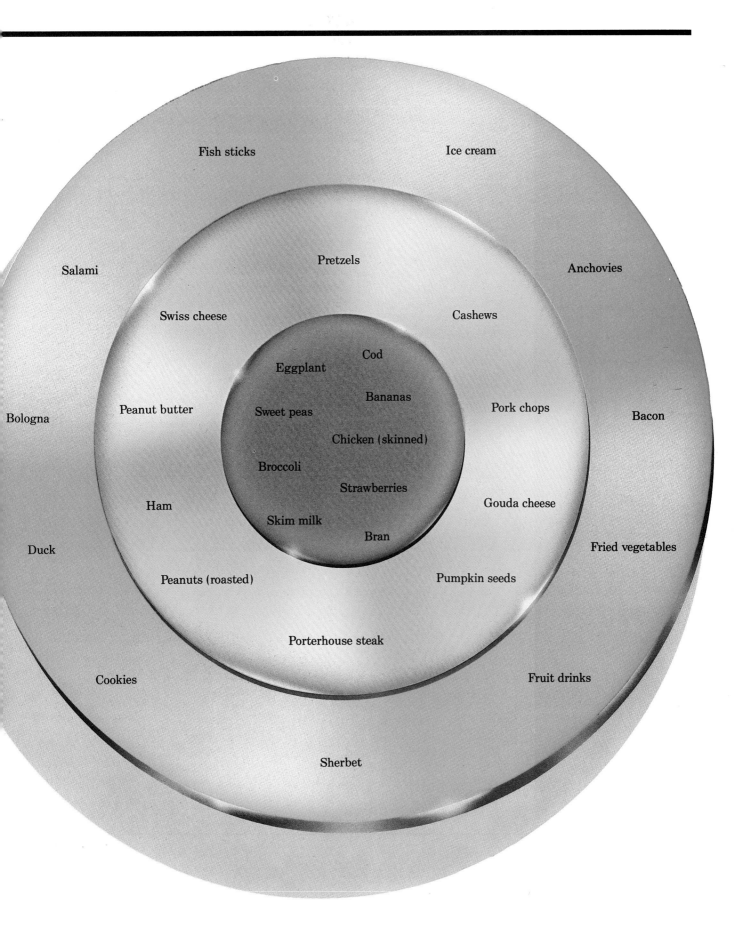

Fish sticks

Ice cream

Pretzels

Salami

Anchovies

Swiss cheese

Cashews

Cod

Eggplant

Bananas

Peanut butter

Sweet peas

Pork chops

Bologna

Chicken (skinned)

Bacon

Broccoli

Strawberries

Ham

Gouda cheese

Skim milk

Duck

Bran

Fried vegetables

Peanuts (roasted)

Pumpkin seeds

Porterhouse steak

Cookies

Fruit drinks

Sherbet

The Ins and Outs of Fiber

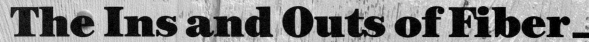

Name this essential nutrient: It's not a vitamin or a mineral, yet it shows up in everything from bulgur to blueberries. It comes in at least 5 different forms. And medical evidence says it can protect us from ills ranging from the merely annoying to the truly life-threatening. The wonder nutrient? Dietary fiber.

Years ago, nutritional scientists thought of dietary fiber the way they once thought of "vitamin B." Supposedly it was a single substance with a single function—to add bulk to the diet and prevent constipation. Now research labs around the world show that there are various forms of fiber, just as there are various kinds of B vitamins. More important, researchers add support to decade-old hypotheses that fiber may help to prevent chronic conditions from overweight to colon cancer. Here's how several common health problems can be helped with fiber.

Overweight. Doctors are recommending bulky, high-fiber foods to overweight people because fiber fills them up but not out. High-fiber foods, such as apples, satisfy the appetite while adding few calories to the daily total.

Hemorrhoids. "A lifetime history of a high-fiber diet is the best way to prevent hemorrhoids, and switching to a high-fiber diet is also the best way to treat many types," says Melvin Bubrick, M.D., a surgeon at Park Nicollet Medical Center in Minneapolis. "People usually feel better within three or four days after starting a high-fiber diet, but it might take them as long as two weeks to adjust," says Dr. Bubrick. "We recommend unprocessed bran and psyllium-based supplements."

Diabetes. Fiber seems to work against diabetes by slowing down the release of sugar into the bloodstream, thereby preventing a sudden, enormous demand for insulin, the hormone that guides sugar molecules to the cells to be burned for fuel.

"Many diabetics don't need insulin. They need a diet program," says James Anderson, M.D., of the University of Kentucky, a recognized pioneer in the treatment of diabetes. Using a high-fiber, ultra-low-fat diet, Dr. Anderson claims that he has been able to reduce the insulin needs of his patients anywhere from 25 to 100 percent, depending on the type of diabetes.

Heart Disease. High cholesterol levels are one of the primary causes of heart disease, and certain kinds of fiber, along with exercise and a low-fat diet, seem to bring cholesterol levels tumbling down. (See "Finding the Fiber You Need" to learn which types have this effect.)

Diverticulosis. Not long ago, the treatment for this disease was a *low*-fiber diet. Now studies show that the reverse might be helpful. A study on animals, conducted in England, suggests that doubling fiber intake could halve the rate of diverticulosis in that country.

Colon Cancer. The National Cancer Institute (NCI) urges everyone to get more fiber in their diets, because they believe that fiber can prevent the disease.

"We feel pretty confident that fiber is involved in the prevention of colon cancer," says Joseph Cullen, Ph.D., of the NCI's Division of Cancer Prevention and Control. "It appears that people who eat more fiber have more protection against colon cancer."

Colon cancer is thought to be triggered by the presence of carcinogens (cancer-causing substances) in the digestive tract. Sometimes the carcinogens are present in food, and sometimes they're produced by intestinal bacteria. Either way, fiber may help the colon empty faster, flushing out the carcinogens before the body can absorb them.

TASTY WAYS TO ADD FIBER TO YOUR DIET

All that good news explains why you may have noticed a surge in the popularity of high-fiber breakfast cereals. Food makers are eager to fortify foods with fiber in hopes of appealing to an increasingly fiber-conscious public.

Here are some other ways to add fiber and flavor to your diet: Leave the peels on apples when you bake them or make applesauce. Roll chicken in corn bran or oat bran for oven baking. Add barley to vegetable soup. Make tostadas with beans instead of beef. Or substitute beans for some or all of the meat in casseroles. Top yogurt with bran, sunflower seeds or chopped apples. Make your own breakfast granola with rolled oats, bran, raisins, slivered almonds and dried fruit. Eat fresh, unpeeled fruit instead of drinking fruit juice. Snack on popcorn. Create desserts from fresh, unpeeled fruit such as peaches and pears. (Fill unpeeled peach halves with cottage cheese and slivered almonds, for example.) Eat potatoes with the skins on. Add cooked beans to tuna salad or pasta salads.

Clearly, there's more to the fiber story than eating bran to keep regular. Working more high-fiber foods into your diet is probably one of the most important things you can do to promote overall good health.

Finding the Fiber You Need

Fiber Type	Probable Functions	Food Sources	
Cellulose	Relieves constipation; counteracts carcinogens in the intestinal tract; modulates glucose; curbs weight gain.	Apples Bran and whole grain cereals Brazil nuts Brussels sprouts Carrots Lima beans	Peanut butter Peanuts Pears Peas Rhubarb Whole wheat bread Whole wheat flour
Pectin	Lowers cholesterol; counters bile acids in the intestinal tract; offers protection against colon cancer and gallstone formation.	Apples Bananas Beets Carrots Okra	Pears Plums Potatoes Strawberries
Gums (mucilages)	Lower cholesterol; modulate glucose levels.	Barley Dried beans Oat bran Oatmeal	Oats Psyllium Rye
Hemicellulose	Relieves constipation; counteracts carcinogens in the intestinal tract; curbs weight gain.	Apples Bananas Beets Bran and whole grain cereals Brussels sprouts	Green beans Lima beans Peas Radishes Sweet corn Whole wheat bread
Lignin	Escorts bile acids and cholesterol out of the intestines; offers protection against colon cancer and gallstone formation.	Apples Bran and whole grain cereals Brazil nuts Cabbage Grapefruit	Peaches Peanuts Pears Peas Strawberries Tomatoes Whole wheat bread

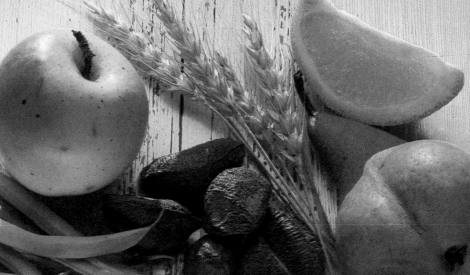

TRENDY NEW FOODS: HOW DO THEY RATE?

Like wide ties and miniskirts, foods go in and out of style. Some foods, like Tofutti, the cholesterol-free ice cream made from soybeans, are totally new commercial concoctions. Others, like phyllo dough and goat's milk cheese, have been around for thousands of years—in other lands.

Serving these trendy new foods may impress your dinner guests. But how do they rate nutritionally? We chose 20 foods at random and evaluated them strictly for their nutritional value—good or bad.

Rating Key

★ ★ ★ ★ Excellent   ★ ★ Fair   X Avoid
    ★ ★ ★ Very good   ★ Enjoy only occasionally

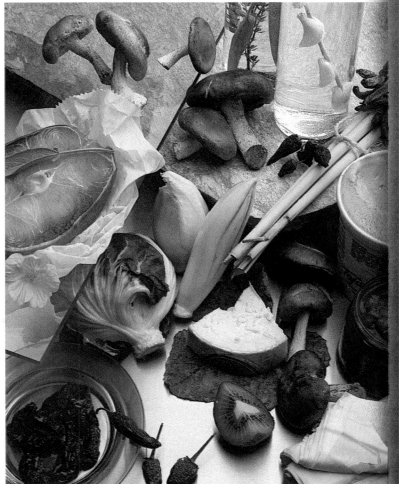

Croissants

Delicate and yummy, to be sure. But these flaky crescent-shaped rolls contain outrageous amounts of butter—and 233 calories per roll. (That's *before* you daub on jam and more butter.)
Rating: ★

Buffalo Wings

Fry chicken wings, soak them in hot sauce, serve them with blue cheese dressing and what do you get? Eighteen percent more fat than unbuffaloed wings: 51 grams of fat and 650 calories per serving, to be exact.
Rating: X

Chevre Cheese

A popular goat's milk cheese, chevre is an excellent source of calcium and a good dietary substitute for cow's milk products for those allergic to them. Best yet, this creamy import is even a little lower in fat than many popular cheeses.
Rating: ★

Monkfish

Thick white fillets of monkfish taste something like lobster when cooked. The nutritional makeup of this fish resembles that of cod—it's a good source of B vitamins and scant amounts of fat or sodium. A great catch!
Rating: ★ ★ ★ ★

Shiitake Mushrooms

These meaty Japanese fungi (available in the U.S. only in their dried form) are so flavorful you can cut way back on salt or other seasonings in soups, stews and other dishes.
Rating: ★ ★ ★

Radicchio

A variety of wild chicory, this red, crinkly salad vegetable is a fair source of vitamin A and vitamin C. It tastes slightly bitter, but pleasantly so.
Rating: ★ ★ ★ ★

Flavored Vinegars

Raspberry, tarragon and basil are among the many fruits, herbs, seeds and spices used to flavor vinegars. Use the flavor-enhanced vinegars to add zest to sauces, marinades and salads—without adding salt or calories.
Rating: ★ ★ ★

Belgian Endive

A versatile vegetable: Toss it into salads, braise and serve it with meat, or roll it up and fill with spreads or dips. This endive has some fiber but is not an outstanding source of any vitamin or mineral.
Rating: ★ ★ ★

Tofutti

This soybean-based frozen dessert has no cholesterol. And it's lactose free. But Tofutti sold in supermarkets (as opposed to its over-the-counter, cone cousin) also has more fat and calories than ice cream, without nearly the amount of calcium.
Rating: ★

Sun-Dried Tomatoes

They're dark and shriveled, but what sun-dried tomatoes lack in looks they make up for in magnificant aroma, rich taste and vitamins C and A. Avoid sun-dried tomatoes that are salted or packed in oil.
Rating: ★ ★ ★ ★

Jambalaya

This is a flavorful Cajun dish that may include shrimp or other seafood, meat, poultry or ham, plus tomatoes. It's a good source of iron, thiamine (vitamin B_1) and niacin.
Rating: ★ ★

Gourmet Mustards

Used in place of fatty spreads such as mayonnaise and Russian dressing, or blended into them, these sauces are a flavorful way to moisten a sandwich. They're available mild or hot, finely or coarsely ground, with many different flavorings.
Rating: ★ ★ ★

Thai Cuisine

Thai cuisine is a Southeast Asian cuisine centered around steamed, stir-fried or braised fish and vegetables, seasoned with fresh coriander, chili peppers, coconut, garlic, limes or lemon grass.
Rating: ★ ★ ★ (provided you go easy on the coconut, a source of saturated fat)

Salsa

This is a super alternative to fatty or sugary sauces, made of chili peppers, tomatoes, onions, fresh coriander leaves, vinegar and corn oil. A staple in Mexican cuisine, it supplies vitamin C, potassium and vitamin A.
Rating: ★ ★ ★ ★

Crayfish

These freshwater crustaceans look like tiny lobsters. They're delicious sauteed, stuffed, or in bisque or other seafood dishes. And don't worry about the cholesterol: There's only 27 milligrams per serving.
Rating: ★ ★

Jicama

Call this a Mexican potato, and pronounce it *he-CA-ma*. Peel it, slice it, dice it and toss it in salads. Or stir-fry, like water chestnuts; a good source of vitamin C.
Rating: ★ ★ ★ ★

Ugli Fruit

Ugli fruit is a cross between an orange and a grapefruit, only misshapen. And it is ugly. But it's an excellent source of vitamin C, even if it's not the prettiest fruit in the world.
Rating: ★ ★ ★ ★

Phyllo

This is a paper-thin, strudellike dough used in Middle Eastern pies and pastries. By itself, the dough is lower in fat and calories than standard crust. But layered with lots of melted butter, its fat content rises dramatically.
Rating: X

Sushi

Sushi may consist of rolled seaweed stuffed with rice and vegetables—or with raw fish. Unfortunately, the fish can harbor a small worm. To be extra-careful, eat only fish with light-colored flesh, and only in reputable restaurants.
Rating: ★ ★ or ★ ★ ★ (depending on ingredients)

Kiwi Fruit

Brown and furry on the outside, sweet and green on the inside, kiwi fruit tastes like a cross between a strawberry and a watermelon. They're a bountiful source of vitamin C, with some iron and potassium.
Rating: ★ ★ ★ ★

Great Cooking Gadgets

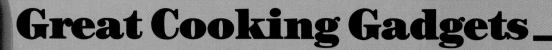

The right tools can change food preparation from a ho-hum chore to a fun-filled adventure. Some gadgets, such as the food processor, are modern precision instruments that do the work of several kitchen helpers with the flick of a switch.

Convenience aside, these kitchen servants also bestow nutritional advantages. Some keep extra fat out of foods; others eliminate the need for added salt by optimizing food's inherent good taste. Most also conserve valuable vitamins and minerals.

Mortar and Pestle

Made of stone, porcelain or wood, this is one of the oldest food tools known. Use it to pulverize seeds, nuts, spices, herbs and garlic. By releasing the full, fresh flavors of those seasonings, cooks often use less salt.

Food Processor

A kitchen helper that performs many tasks—fast. Slice or shred pounds of fruit or vegetables in minutes. Process meat or fish into a pâté without adding eggs or cream, or make cream soups without thickeners.

Meat Thermometer

It monitors the internal temperature of meat to prevent undercooking (which can trigger food-borne illness) or overcooking (which destroys flavor, texture and heat-soluble nutrients).

Gravy Separator

Fat rises to the top of hot broth in this 1- to 2-cup vessel. Pour off the grease and what's left is a low-fat stock, sauce or gravy.

No-Stick Fry Pan

The special finish on the inner surface of this pan allows for frying or sauteeing without using cooking fat. The food will not burn to the pan.

Fish Poacher

Simmered in liquid in this oblong saucepan, fish stays moist and flavorful without fat or salt. Aromatic herbs such as dill or rosemary and garnishes such as garlic and onions are delicious additions to the simmering liquid.

Pasta Machine

Whether hand cranked or electrically driven, a pasta machine produces light, tasty noodles. Add carrot puree for added vitamin A or pureed broccoli for vitamin C.

Pressure Cooker

By increasing the air pressure and so raising water's boiling point, this device cooks food faster. (The hotter the water, the faster food gets done.) As a result, healthful dishes that usually cook for hours—bean soups, chicken stock, pot roast or squash— become convenient to prepare.

Knife Sharpener

Sharp knives allow you to slice meat and vegetables more thinly, shortening cooking time and conserving nutrients.

Terrine

An oval or rectangular ceramic ovenproof dish with a lid, a terrine is great for combining seasoned, minced vegetables, seafood, poultry and grains into hearty, make-ahead loaves.

Salad Spinner

Centrifugal force gets rid of water droplets, which can leach vitamins from greens and make them (and berries) soggy. Dressing clings better to dry greens, so you can use less and save calories.

Microwave Oven

Microwaves cook by feverishly bouncing food molecules against each other, generating friction and heat. This shorter, low-water method of cooking helps retain vitamins and minerals in food.

3

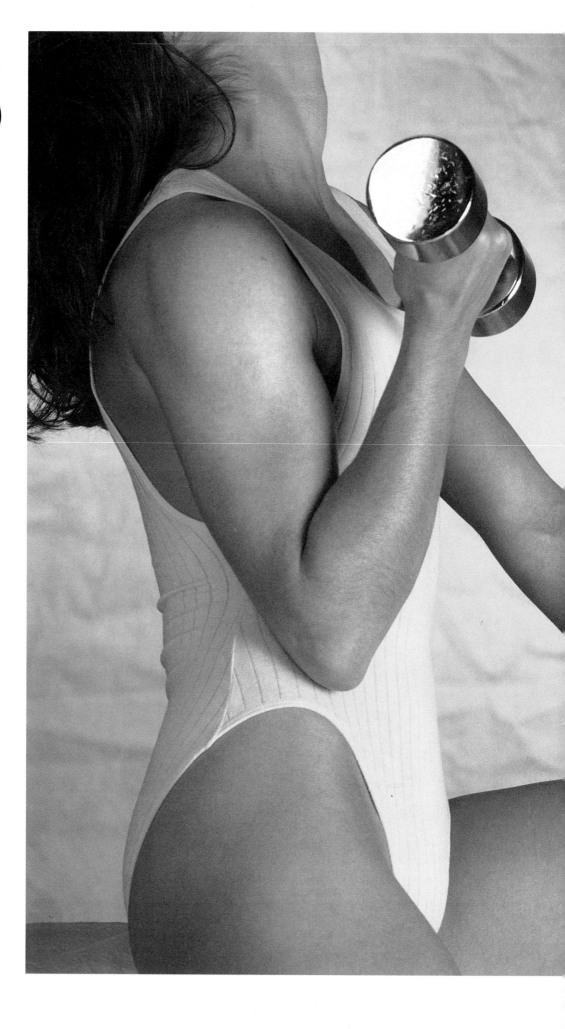

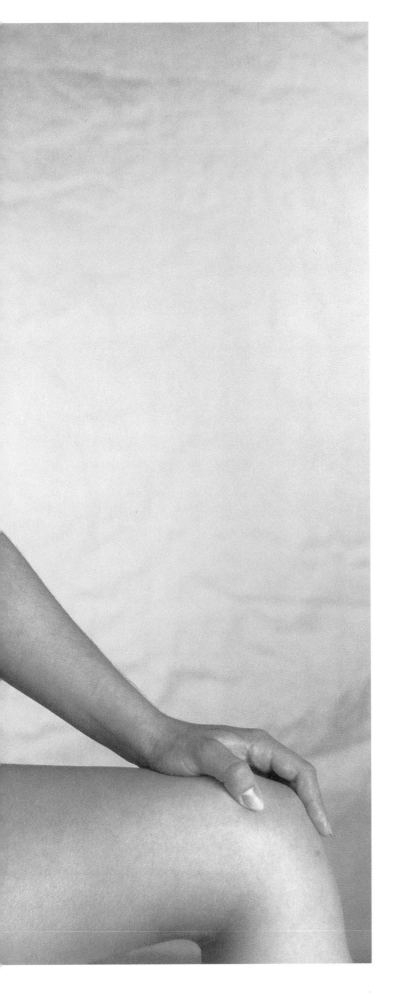

Mastering Fitness

Machines wear out with use.
But your body will grow
stronger if you work it hard.

Have you ever watched Magic Johnson execute a flying dunk and wished you were half as graceful and athletic as he is? Or do the mere words "50-yard dash" strike terror in your heart?

Some people love to exercise. Others hate it. Most of us fall somewhere in between. Perhaps you've honestly tried to exercise regularly but felt sore after an aerobics class or two. Or you got bored and discouraged after a few early-morning jaunts on the jogging trail. Or you're too busy to exercise. Or you think you're too old. Or too overweight. Or just not the athletic type.

Perhaps you've heard that exercise is healthy but you want to be sure you're doing it right, to avoid injury.

If you have a lot of questions—and mixed emotions—about exercise, you're not alone. Exercise dropouts, sports novices and lifetime armchair quarterbacks alike all wonder at one time or another, "Does exercise really do people any good? Should *I* exercise? What kind of exercise is best? Do I have to run to get in shape? How long and how often should I work out? How do I start? How can I keep from getting bored?"

We hope to clear up the confusion once and for all and launch you on a fitness program that'll begin to pay off in just a couple of weeks and continue to pay off for the rest of your life, no matter what your age. Because exercise is *definitely* good for you. And you don't have to be a natural athlete, a marathon runner or a hard-core jock to benefit.

And while exercise is beneficial for your health, it also should be *fun*! In fact, exercising for health and health alone is like eating food for calories and nutrients alone. You miss the pleasure of the experience. So above all, you must pick activities you enjoy. That doesn't necessarily mean you have to engage in thrill sports such as scuba diving or downhill skiing to get your kicks. After all, recreation of any kind is daring if you've never done it before. Even something as simple as

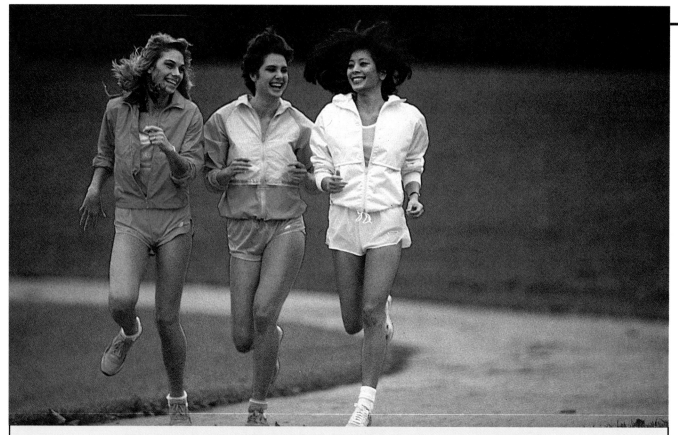

Using Your Heartbeat to Increase Fitness

When world-class athletes wake up in the morning, often the first thing they do is take their pulse. Why? Your heart rate—the number of times your heart beats in a minute—is a good indicator of how efficiently blood is being pumped through the circulatory system. It's also a good indicator of your overall health and level of fitness. World-class athletes, for instance, can have resting heart rates as low as 36 to 40, compared with the average person's 60 to 100 beats per minute.

The resting heart rate is just that—a measurement of how often your heart beats when you are making no particular demands on your body. To determine your resting heart rate, take your pulse by counting the beats for 1 minute on the artery located on your wrist, below the heel of your thumb. Be sure to wrap your middle finger around your wrist to feel the pulse, as the thumb has a pulse of its own.

Record your resting heart rate in a diary or on your calendar for several weeks to find what's normal for you.

Gradually, through an exercise program, you'll see your resting heart rate drop. Your heart will grow stronger and won't have to beat as often.

During exercise you will get this benefit by working your heart hard enough to increase its muscle mass and aerobic capacity. In order to do that, you've got to push your heart to beat to the training heart rate, which is at least 60 percent of its maximum capacity.

To calculate your training heart rate, subtract your age in years from 220 (for men) or 226 (for women). Now calculate 60 percent of this figure. This is your minimum training heart rate.

For example, if you are a 40-year-old woman, you would subtract 40 from 226, giving you a base of 186. A training rate would be 60 percent of that number or 186 times 0.60, which equals 111 beats per minute. If you want to train more vigorously, increase the 60 percent to 85 percent, but never exceed that percentage of your heart's capacity. It leads to exhaustion and possible injury.

walking can be highly exhilarating. Walkers rhapsodize about the thrill of being close to nature—hearing the geese call as they arrow southward, or watching a spectacular sunset. At the same time, walking happens to be one of the best exercises anyone can do.

But first, let's set the record straight on what exercise can and cannot do for you.

THE HEALTH DIVIDENDS OF REGULAR EXERCISE

Everyone knows that exercise helps you control your weight—or reduce it—by burning calories. But did you know that a good workout can help the overwrought as well as the overweight? Some researchers claim that by triggering the release of natural opiates (bodily substances that help you feel relaxed), brisk exercise can enable you to bend, not break, under stress. Feeling a little blue? Anxious for no good reason? Fidgety and fretful? A run around the block or a pickup game of volleyball can dispel worry and lift your mood. That's probably why kids have so much fun.

Exercise has tangible health effects, too. Physical activity increases the flow of calcium and other minerals into your bones, strengthening your skeleton. If you don't exercise, the opposite may occur: Your bones may automatically lose minerals and become as brittle and breakable as a china teacup, especially if you're a woman past menopause.

Exercise also strengthens muscles in your abdomen and upper legs, which can then share the workload otherwise carried by your lower back. Thus, exercise prevents chronic low back pain for many people. Regular physical activity can also ward off much of the muscle weakness and joint pain associated with arthritis.

The really *big* news, though, is what exercise can do for your heart. Thirty years of medical research have shown that your heart probably can't stay healthy without exercise. A lifetime spent sitting on your duff is just as real a risk factor for heart disease as smoking cigarettes or developing high blood pressure. Con-versely, regular physical activity— walking, gardening or other forms of physical work and play—may reduce your risk of heart attack by up to 40 percent. Part of the reason that exercise is so good for your heart (and the arteries that feed it) is that vigorous activity reduces circulating levels of blood fats called triglycer-ides and LDL (low-density lipoprotein) cholesterol, both of which clog blood vessels and cut off the oxygen supply to your heart. At the same time, exercise helps your heart thrive by raising levels of HDL (high-density lipoprotein) cholesterol, which is good for your heart.

If all these health dividends aren't enough to propel you from your easy chair, consider that exer-cise also helps reduce your risk of developing high blood pressure (an important factor in whether you develop heart disease or have a stroke). Exercise also regulates blood sugar levels and therefore may help control diabetes or even prevent it.

Exercise keeps your batteries charged, increasing the amount of work you can do without getting tired and out of breath. And exercise gives you flexibility and coordi-nation, cutting your chances for an accident.

We wish we could say that exercise also guarantees additional years of life. Maybe it does, but the evidence isn't conclusive. What *is* clear is that exercise definitely adds life to your years, because many of the changes we blame on old age— weight gain, fatigue, stiff joints, weak muscles, angina, high blood pressure and so forth—may not be inevitable. They're the price we pay for living in a world of elevators, cars and golf carts. We're built for action, and we should be hitting the trails instead of sitting on our tails.

"As a species, humans have pursued cerebral fitness at the expense of physical fitness," says Per-Olof Astrand, M.D., a Swedish scientist who is to exercise physiology what the Wright brothers were to aviation. "Exercise isn't optional—it's manda-tory for a healthful life. Yet as chil-dren we are repeatedly told, 'Don't jump on the furniture. Don't climb trees. Don't get your clothes dirty. Go watch TV and be quiet.' So as

A Road Test for Your Heart

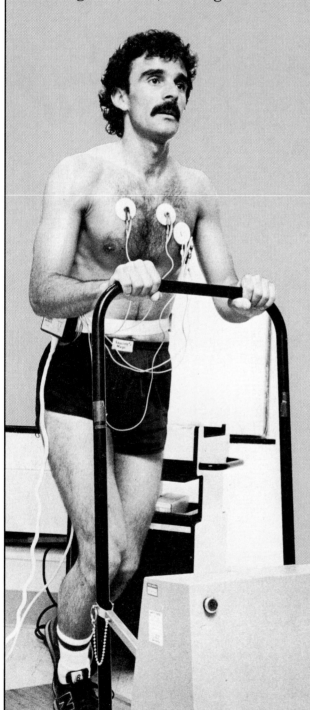

If you're over 40 and beginning a strenuous exercise program, your doctor will probably ask you to take an exercise stress test. Several electrodes are attached to your chest and other spots and hooked up to a machine that prints out an electrocardiogram (ECG) showing information about your heartbeat and heart rhythm.

This information tells your doctor how your heart functions under physical stress (something that doesn't show up on a resting ECG). One of the most important measurements recorded is called the ST segment. It shows whether your heart muscle is getting enough oxygen while you exercise.

Like most tests, the exercise stress test isn't perfect. Studies show that it can occasionally fail to reveal existing heart disease, thus giving the green light to people who really should proceed with exercise cautiously. Conversely, a stress test can sometimes give a false indication of heart problems where none exist, thus giving the red light to people who could exercise safely. Doctors urge that the stress test always be considered *along with* a thorough medical history and other tests for heart disease, to help interpret the results.

The test is most useful in people over 40 who have known risk factors for heart disease (such as a family history of heart disease, high blood pressure, high cholesterol or a history of smoking) or who suffer symptoms of heart disease (chest pain, breathlessness, fatigue, palpitations, indigestion).

A positive stress test (indicating the possibility of heart disease) doesn't automatically rule out exercise. Rather, the results can help your doctor to prescribe an exercise program that is safe for you, given your individual circumstances. Jim Fixx, the noted runner and author, might be alive today if he had taken a stress test to analyze why he was having chest pain, especially since he'd once been overweight and smoked heavily, took up jogging late in life and came from a family whose members suffered heart problems.

children we learn that physical activity is socially unacceptable—and we grow up into sedentary adults," Dr. Astrand explains.

SCARED TO DEATH OF EXERCISE?

"Runner Dies while Jogging"

Headlines like that leave many people skeptical about the health benefits of exercise. They needn't worry. The risk of sudden death during or after exercise is very small, very preventable—and heavily outweighed by the long-term health benefits.

"More people die of sudden cardiac death during sedentary activities like watching TV than while running or pursuing other strenuous sports," according to Terence Kavanagh, M.D., medical director of the Toronto Rehabilitation Centre and a doctor famed for training heart attack veterans to run in the Boston Marathon. "Medical evidence shows that people who die of a heart attack during exercise would have died soon anyway, whether they exercised or not, because of preexisting— and sometimes hidden—heart disease," Dr. Kavanagh told an audience of physicians at the Masters Games Sportsmedicine Symposium in Toronto.

Talk about deaths among runners, and the name Jim Fixx comes up in conversation. His is an instructive case.

"It's important to keep in mind that Jim Fixx started to exercise late in life and had quite a few risk factors for heart disease—he'd been a heavy smoker, had been overweight—and he had refused a stress test [to diagnose heart disease] despite chest pain and other warning signs," comments Canadian physician Robert McKelvie, M.D.

"Our studies suggest that half the people who drop dead while jogging had complained to their spouses about symptoms or had even made appointments to see their doctors and then went out and jogged their last mile," says Paul D. Thompson, M.D., a cardiologist and

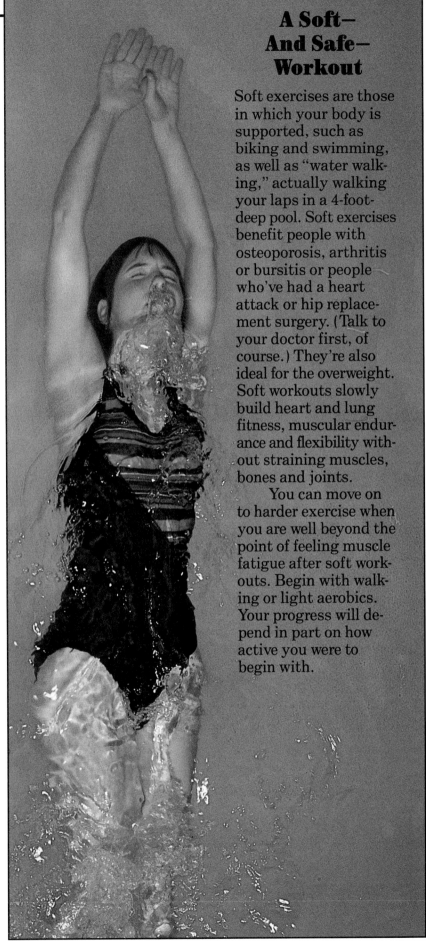

A Soft— And Safe— Workout

Soft exercises are those in which your body is supported, such as biking and swimming, as well as "water walking," actually walking your laps in a 4-foot-deep pool. Soft exercises benefit people with osteoporosis, arthritis or bursitis or people who've had a heart attack or hip replacement surgery. (Talk to your doctor first, of course.) They're also ideal for the overweight. Soft workouts slowly build heart and lung fitness, muscular endurance and flexibility without straining muscles, bones and joints.

You can move on to harder exercise when you are well beyond the point of feeling muscle fatigue after soft workouts. Begin with walking or light aerobics. Your progress will depend in part on how active you were to begin with.

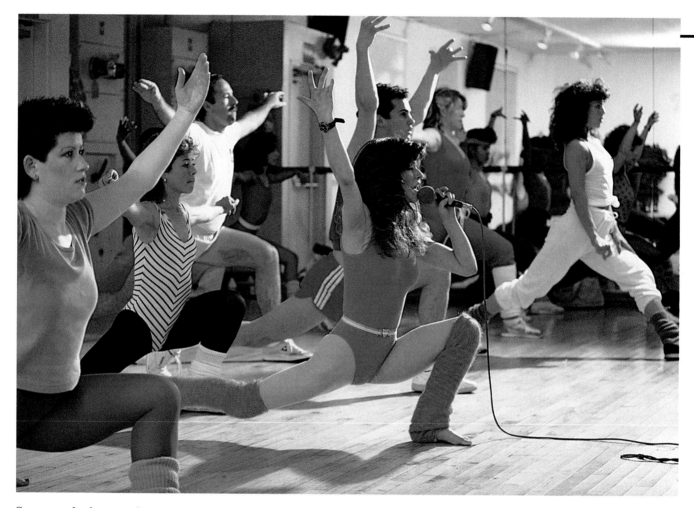

Some people shy away from aerobics classes because they feel they have no dance talent. With a little patience and some individual attention, though, anyone can enjoy aerobics, according to Molly Fox, of Molly Fox's Heavenly Bodies exercise studio in New York.

"Look for an uncrowded class (with 25 or fewer participants) and an instructor who can give you individual attention—*showing* you how to place your feet correctly, extend your arms, lift your legs and breathe when you should," Ms. Fox explains. "If you have trouble keeping in step with the others, stand in the back and imitate someone who looks like they know what they're doing. And most of all, don't take your 'mistakes' too seriously." After all, you're not auditioning for the Folies-Bergère.

associate professor of medicine at Brown University.

Many doctors say that when they tell people to exercise, they also prescribe a hefty dose of common sense. If you experience any warning signs of heart trouble during exertion—chest pain, excessive breathlessness, indigestion, heart palpitations or fatigue—stop exercising. And see your doctor as soon as possible. If you feel well, chances are you have little to worry about.

"The fact is, millions of people jog without dying while doing it," assures Dr. Thompson. "If you feel perfectly well, you have an extremely small chance of having a heart attack during exercise."

MIX FITNESS WITH PLEASURE

With worry banished, you now can choose a sport that suits your personal or social needs. Pick an

activity you enjoy, and you'll still be exercising 20 years from now.

"Few people exercise solely for the health benefits," Dr. Thompson says. "People may start to exercise for their health. But those who continue to exercise do so for pleasure, recognition or some other equally important psychological or social need.

"When people ask what type of exercise is the best, I tell them, 'The best exercise is what *you* want to do.' Keep in mind that what makes you happy may be entirely different from what makes other people happy," continues Dr. Thompson. "For example, bird-watching would bore me to death. But for people who enjoy it, bird-watching is a great way to do lots of walking."

"I took up bird-watching recently," says Dr. Astrand, "and it's the perfect hobby for me because I can combine it not only with walking but also with jogging and cycling."

So Dr. Astrand recommends

that people combine exercise with a hobby. "If you like photography, take your camera with you. Or go berry picking." He feels that tying exercise to a nature hobby enhances the pleasure by making exercise three-dimensional, adding appeal for people who wouldn't ordinarily exercise.

"Exercise should also be convenient," points out Dr. Thompson. "For example, chopping wood burns a lot of calories and is great exercise. But for someone who has no ax, no woodlot and no wood stove, chopping wood would not be practical."

Personality is another factor, he says. "Are you people oriented? Jog with a group or join an aerobics class. If you're competitive by nature, compete."

"But," adds Dr. Astrand, "you don't *have to* compete."

"Competition can give some people the recognition they need, the payback that motivates them to keep going," says Laurence Hewick, Ph.D., a running enthusiast who used his management expertise to organize a marathon race at the first annual Masters Games in Toronto. "But participation in itself is rewarding. So I plan to organize more 5-kilometer and 10-kilometer races—corporate runs, family runs and so forth—so that more folks can win gold, silver and bronze medals. A majority of everyday runners want to compete—but not as elite [highly trained, serious] runners."

While running is economical in terms of time and effort (you work a lot of muscles in a short period of time), it is by no means the only way or the best way to exercise.

"Running is not essential for human survival," remarks Dr. Astrand. "I visited the Kalahari Bushmen in Africa. And I never once saw a Bushman run. I did see them walk extremely fast, however. Statements like that don't make me very popular with running enthusiasts. But the fact remains, walking is just as good an exercise as running is—it just takes you a little longer to get where you're going.

"So walk your dog even if you don't have one," quips Dr. Astrand. "I also recommend swimming, cycling, dancing, rowing or cross-country skiing . . . not fishing, riding a golf cart or horseback riding, where the fish, cart or horse do all the work."

YOUR PACE OR MINE?

Sold on the benefits of getting into shape, but still confused about how much exercise you need?

"Keep exercise simple," Dr. Thompson says. "In some ways, I think we as health professionals have overcomplicated exercise. Kids know how to exercise and no one gives them elaborate formulas or teaches them how to be active. They just do it."

Exercise physiologists—people who make a living figuring out how the human body works best—say that the body especially thrives on physical activity that uses the large muscles of the body, those found in your arms and legs. And we should exercise three times a week for 30 minutes at a crack, doing something that raises the heart rate to about 75 percent of its maximum. (Maximum heart rate is approximately 220 minus your age. If numbers bewilder you or you can't be bothered taking your pulse, just exercise intensely enough to make you slightly out of breath but not so breathless that you can't carry on a conversation, suggests Dr. Thompson.)

Dr. Astrand warns, "Don't be a slave to a stopwatch. Testing for VO_2 max [total body oxygen consumption] and other clinical measurements of fitness is fine for people who are highly competitive or fascinated by numbers. But for most of us, the important thing is to just get out and *do* it."

"People sometimes expect their doctor to prescribe exercise and spell out exactly what to do, when and for how long," comments Dr. Thompson. "But look at people who swim, jog or cycle a lot. They don't do it by formula—they mold exercise to their life."

You should learn, however, to know when you've had enough, so that you avoid injury and fatigue.

"Never exercise so hard that you feel bad afterward," say Lenore R. Zohman, M.D., and Albert A. Kattus, M.D., in their book *The Cardiologists' Guide to Fitness and Health through*

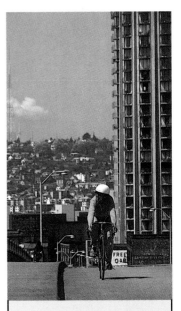

Jog 'n' Job

Run to work. (Or ride your bike, if possible.) It's a great way to guarantee you'll exercise. Carry your papers and personal items in a lightweight, waterproof backpack. Keep a week's worth of clean clothes at the office. Sponge off when you arrive. Or run one way only—home—and then shower.

A Sensible Exercise Plan for Weekend Athletes

Do you try to make up for your sedentary job by playing 3 hours of tennis on Saturday afternoon or jogging 10 miles on Saturday *and* Sunday? Then do you drag your aching muscles and joints to the office on Monday morning feeling like you fought a war—single-handedly? Bryant Stamford, Ph.D., from the exercise physiology lab at the University of Louisville School of Medicine, designed this walk/jog program to bring weekend athletes up to fitness in 3 to 5 months, depending on their age. Sure, it's slow. But by not overstressing your joints, you'll avoid the aches and pains that tempt many weekend athletes to give up sports entirely.

Weekend	Distance per session (miles)	Intensity (for people under age 35) per session (ratio of walking paces to jogging paces)		Intensity (for people over age 35) per session (ratio of walking paces to jogging paces)	
1	½	50	50	75	25
2	¾	50	50	75	25
3	1	50	50	75	25
4	1¼	50	50	75	25
5	1½	50	50	75	25
6	1¾	50	50	75	25
7	2	50	50	75	25
8	2¼	50	50	75	25
9	2½	50	50	75	25
10	2¾	50	50	75	25
11	3	50	50	75	25
12	3	50	100	50	50
13	3	50	200	50	70
14	3	all jog		50	90
15	3	all jog		50	110
16	3	all jog		50	130
17	3	all jog		50	150
18	3	all jog		50	170
19	3	all jog		50	190
20	3	all jog		all jog	

NOTE: If you're not at all active when starting this program, Dr. Stamford recommends slowing down the intensity buildup by half. In other words, the under-35 athlete would increase the jogging paces by only 25 per weekend (starting at the 12th weekend), instead of 50, until he's up to 200 jogging paces. The over-35 athlete would increase the jogging paces by only 10 per weekend (starting at the 13th weekend) instead of 20.

Exercise. "You should feel good for 15 to 20 minutes after you stop and then energetic and invigorated. If you're exercising correctly, the rest of the day should go better than if you hadn't exercised."

It's also important to skip a day between workouts or alternate easy days with hard days, according to Douglas B. Clement, M.D., and Jack E. Taunton, M.D., co-directors of the British Columbia Sportsmedicine Clinic in Vancouver, Canada. Resting or alternating prevents injury by allowing the muscles to rest and adapt to the workload.

ON YOUR MARK, GET SET, GO SLOWLY

"It's easy to get people to start to exercise," says Margo Walsh, an exercise physiologist at the Duke University Medical Center in Durham, North Carolina. "The tough part is getting them to stick with it.

"We find that people who begin exercise slowly are more likely to continue because they're less likely to experience pain and soreness. And less pain means less injury—a leading reason that people quit exercising," Ms. Walsh explains.

"Walking is a great exercise for beginners," says Dr. Thompson. "Walk a while, then jog the distance between two telephone poles. Walk a while longer, then jog the distance between two telephone poles and so forth. That's how you progress."

Jane Katz, Ed.D., a competitive swimmer, teacher and author of three books on swimming for fitness, including *The W.E.T. Workout,* says, "Beginners should start with something they know they can do and work up. Start by jogging in place, then jog a distance. Start by lifting your feet 6 inches off the floor, then lift them 12 inches. If you take an aerobics class, join a beginner class, stretching classes or yoga classes.

"And don't expect overnight results," she adds. "You didn't get out of shape in a week, and you're not going to get back into shape in a week."

When *can* you expect to experience some benefits?

Anywhere from two weeks to three months. Until you actually begin to feel thinner, stronger and more energetic, a simple reward system may help you to keep going, according to Gary deVoss, Ph.D., a psychologist with Optimal Performance Associates in San Diego.

"The first two weeks are the hardest," says Dr. deVoss. "So reward yourself immediately and often. When you come home from exercise class, walk past the dirty dishes and take a luxurious bubble bath. Don't do the housework out of guilt and omit the reward, or you establish a negative association—and stop exercising. Or sit down and relax with your favorite snack or beverage. Make rewards an intrinsic part of your program.

"If you still hate to exercise, reevaluate your reward system. Or choose a new exercise. That'll keep you going until you begin to enjoy exercise for the sake of exercise alone."

Dr. deVoss says you can train yourself to love exercise by adopting a technique used by many athletes.

"To enhance your awareness of the internal rewards of getting fit, write down your pleasurable feelings after exercise," he suggests. "Comments such as 'I feel so much lighter, as though I could jump over the moon'; 'I never realized how great it feels to sweat'; or 'My heart actually feels stronger' reinforce the process—and keep you coming back for more."

EXCUSES, EXCUSES

"I'd like to exercise in the morning, but it's hard to get up early."

"I'd like to exercise at noon, but I often have meetings and can't get away."

"I'd like to exercise after work, but my family expects dinner to be ready by 6:00 P.M."

"I'd like to work out in the evening, but my spouse wants to spend that time with me."

Sound familiar? Lack of time is probably the most common reason people don't exercise. To find time, sit down and account for your day minute by minute, says Dr. deVoss. And then make some changes: Ask your spouse to cook dinner three nights a week or cooperate in some other way. And don't feel guilty about taking time to do something good for yourself.

"Make exercise a business appointment with your body," says Dr. Katz. "Write it on your calendar in ink. If you're supposed to get together with someone for business, invite them to go for a swim or a tennis game and talk business in the steam room.

"Personally, I know my day goes better if I've been in the water," she adds.

"Finding time to exercise is the hardest part of any sport," concedes David Challinor, Ph.D., a competitive rower and head of the science division of the Smithsonian Institution in Washington. But if a busy guy like David can find the time, so can you. "I row when I can—before work, after work or on my lunch hour," he explains.

Lunch hours are a valuable and underused opportunity to exercise, leaving evenings free to spend with your family. Dr. Hewick comments, "In many companies, the traditional 'businessman's lunch' has been replaced by the businessman's or businesswoman's run. Or tennis set. Or racquetball game. Even if you exercise by yourself, working out at lunchtime gives you a chance to take stock of things. If you ask managers or executives if their decision-making ability is better after they've sweated things out than if they went out for a big meal and a couple of drinks, nine out of ten will say yes. The overweight vice president watching his or her colleagues jog from the executive-suite window won't be around too

If you're exercising hard and maintaining your proper weight, you're probably getting enough calories, vitamins and minerals. Be aware, however, that potassium, magnesium and zinc are lost in perspiration. Moreover, if you're a vegetarian, a woman or a dieter, nutrient losses or limited food choices call for special care. (Any supplements listed here are recommendations, not prescriptions. Take them only with the approval and supervision of your doctor.)

The Exerciser's Diet

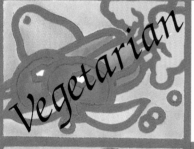

Vegetarian

Because it can be hard for vegetarians to get enough iron, they should try to eat iron-rich foods such as sunflower seeds, almonds, broccoli, spinach, lima beans, peas, raisins, prunes and dried apricots. Those who are pure vegans (who eschew eggs and dairy products) may require vitamin B_{12} supplements.

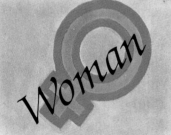

Woman

Women exercisers may require extra amounts of the B vitamins riboflavin and thiamine, as well as iron, zinc and copper. For riboflavin and thiamine, eat plenty of beef or chicken liver, beef kidney, navy beans and brewer's yeast. The liver also helps to provide much-needed iron. Snacking on sunflower seeds may help keep zinc levels high.

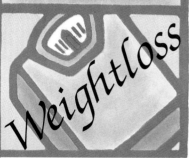

Weightloss

People who are dieting *and* exercising have special needs. They, too, require B vitamins, but must be careful to rely on low-calorie sources such as beef broth, cottage cheese, mushrooms, tuna (packed in water), asparagus, chicken white meat and fish such as bass and swordfish. Because most foods high in zinc are also high in calories, ask your doctor if you should take zinc supplements.

much longer—one way or the other."

Even if Phys. Ed. became a required course for an MBA degree, some would-be exercisers would still have one last hurdle to clear: self-consciousness. Many first-timers are bound to feel they're too awkward to exercise, or too slow, or too old.

To overcome such unproductive thoughts, Dr. deVoss suggests that people adopt the rationale that there's bound to be someone else who's in worse shape than you are. And if there isn't? What if you *are* the heaviest or most uncoordinated person in the group? Well, you won't be for long! Think of how much you'll improve if you stick with it.

Another trick that Dr. deVoss says works against self-conscious thoughts is exaggerating your fears to the point of absurdity.

"Say you're jogging down the street thinking that people are looking out their windows, laughing at you because you're so out of shape. How many people are peering at you? Fifty? A hundred? *A thousand?* And who has time to stand at their window and laugh at joggers, anyway?"

Dr. deVoss says it also helps to buddy up with someone who'll encourage you to exercise together.

A close second to the fat-person-jogging-down-the-street-while-the-neighbors-titter scenario is enrolling in an exercise class full of people who look like they don't need to exercise at all. Don't ask yourself, "Is this an exercise class or a beauty pageant?" or, "What am I doing here?" And no matter what, don't run home and eat two pieces of chocolate cake in discouragement.

"If you take a closer look, you'll see that not everyone in aerobics classes is in perfect shape," says Molly Fox, of Molly Fox's Heavenly Bodies, an exercise studio in New York City. "If you feel self-conscious, take a position in the back row. If it's too painful to look at yourself in the mirror, don't look in the mirror. If you're top-heavy or carry a little too much weight around your middle, you may want to wear a jazzy over-size T-shirt over your leotard. If you're hippy, try wearing bright parachute-style dance pants. And remember, there's no such thing as the perfect body."

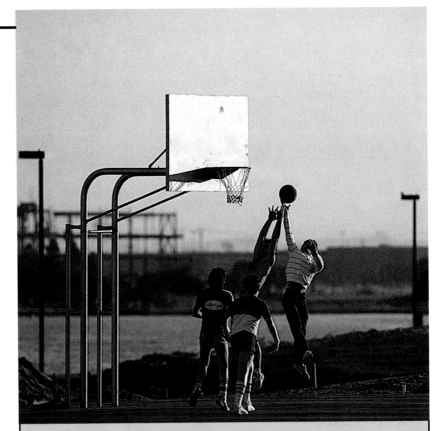

The Joys of the Pickup Game

Slam-dunk your way to health. Fly a saucer for fitness. Volley for VO$_2$ max. Sound like fun ways to work out? You bet. Frequent, impromptu games of basketball, Frisbee or volleyball—or any other running-jumping-throwing game—can round out your exercise program nicely. Because if you love what you're doing, you'll do it with zest—and get a good workout. Pickup games are also a great way to unwind after work with neighbors or co-workers—and live out your fantasies as an ace wide receiver or other star athlete.

Touch football, badminton, soccer, ice hockey, water polo and greased watermelon races also make good pickup games. Where to play? In city parks, ponds and pools; schoolyards after hours, church or community gymnasiums; company parking lots; driveways and backyards—anywhere people congregate to recreate.

Dr. Astrand says: "Getting in shape is like quitting smoking or drinking less or taking any other positive health step. Don't postpone it. Do it *now*."

And have fun!

Masters of Fitness

Call it *Jeux des Maîtres*. Or *Juegos Veteranos*. Or Olympics for people over 25—and up to 80. The first Masters Games took place in Toronto, Canada, in August 1985—a 22-ring circus of competition and fun for born-again athletes, competing in sports as thrilling as boardsailing or as underrated as badminton. Also competing in basketball, canoeing, cycling, swimming, tennis, rowing and ice hockey, more than 12,000 athletes from all over the world participated and had a ball. Here, 6 Masters Games athletes share their thoughts about lifetime sports and fitness.

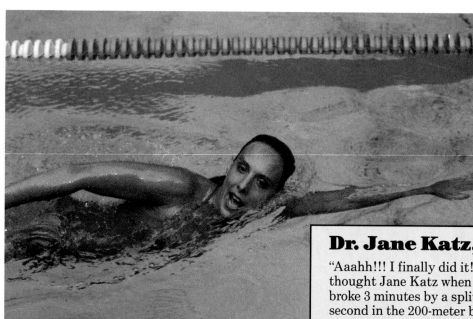

Dr. Jane Katz, 43, Swimmer

"Aaahh!!! I finally did it!" So thought Jane Katz when she broke 3 minutes by a split second in the 200-meter back-stroke and won a gold medal in her division.

"It's only a fraction of a second," Jane says, "but it's a big hurdle. It proves that you *can* get better as you get older. And I think swimming is the ideal lifetime sport for just about anyone."

Ed Benham, 78, Runner

"I'd rather run than do anything else," says Ed, a retired jockey who started running—and competing—at the age of 72. "I meet wonderful people when I compete, and running gives me something to look forward to."

Ed holds just about every world's record for running in his age group, and won the 10-kilometer race at the Masters Games in 42:45.00.

"See what older people can do?" quips Ed confidently. "I'm healthier than ever—haven't sneezed in years. And my blood pressure is normal. That's unusual for someone my age."

Mary Ayer, 60, Tennis Player

"I played a total of 1 match at the Masters Games—my opponent happened to be a former coach for Martina Navratilova and beat me 6-2, 6-0," Mary says good-naturedly. "But I had a lot of fun anyway, because I entered the games for the primary purpose of participating and meeting other tennis players."

Now there's a good sport!

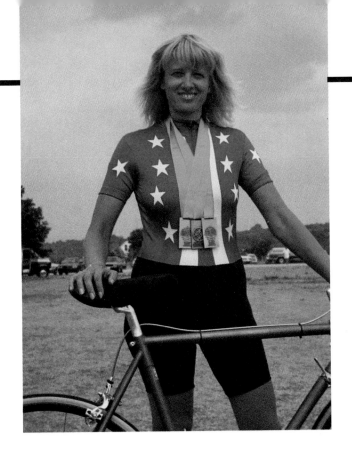

Dottie Saling, 41, Cyclist

Dottie was totally surprised when she finished a close second in the 47-kilometer road race. She hadn't expected the big hill that loomed midcourse.

"I hate hills," Dottie says. "But I just pedaled all the harder and went for broke. And when I reached the crest, I realized I was alone."

Another cyclist eventually caught up to—and passed—her. But the near victory whetted her appetite for further competition. A cyclist since the age of 13, Dottie left cycling for a few years to raise a family. Since she resumed training, she's as enthusiastic—and fit—as ever.

Dr. David Challinor, 65, Rower

From March to December David, who was formerly on the Harvard varsity crew, rows an average of 5 miles a day on the Potomac. In his travels for the Smithsonian Institution, David's rowed all over the world—on the Thames, on the Nile and on the rivers of Rangoon—"wherever I can find a river and a boat," he says.

David's passion for rowing peaked at the Masters Games: His crew won 3 events and took 3rd place in another.

"The camaraderie among rowers is great—probably what I enjoy most about the sport," David says. "And I feel better when I row. It helps me think more clearly."

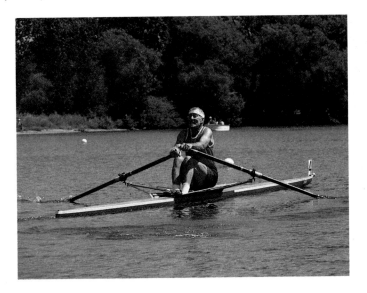

LeRoy Ellis, 45, Basketball Player

"NBA basketball is definitely a young man's game," says LeRoy, formerly with the LA Lakers, Philadelphia 76ers and Baltimore (now Washington) Bullets. "You have to run fast and jump high, and it's highly competitive. But Masters basketball is *fun*—everyone is the same age and at the same level of fitness. Of course, I have a slight edge because I'm 6'11" and played professionally for years. And our team—East Bank Saloon—won 7 games in 8 days. But mainly, I play for the exercise—twice a week when I can. Basketball will probably always be a part of my life."

41

4

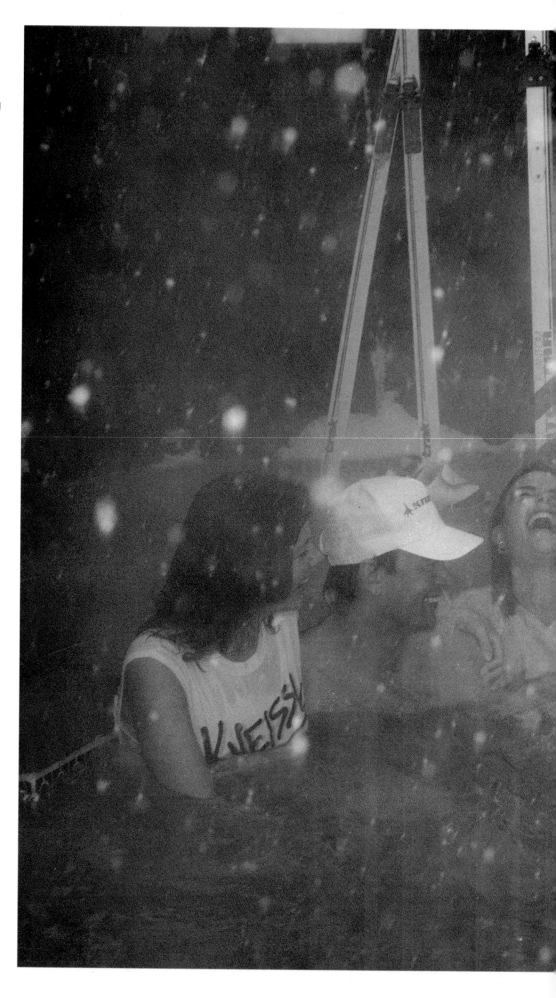

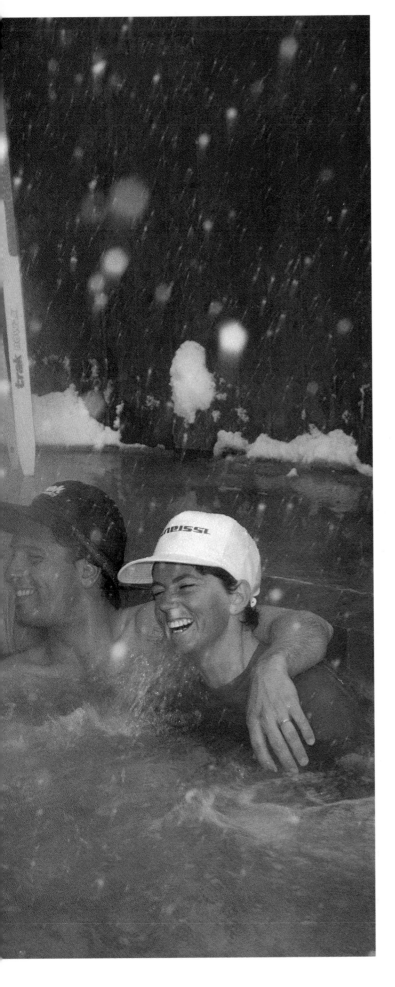

Mastering Happiness

Can you capture the bluebird of happiness? The fun is in the trying, say the experts.

It's time to get serious about happiness. That's what the scientists tell us. Their latest studies say that if we're too hostile, too lonely or just plain too miserable too much of the time, these feelings may damage our health, even cut short our lives.

Ever since the great stress researcher, the late Hans Selye, M.D., began looking into the health effects of stress half a century ago, it's been clear that inescapable suffering can damage immune systems, creating vulnerability to illness.

Even those most skeptical of the connection between negative feelings and ill health are likely to find the latest scientific work eerily convincing.

In one study of 227 people, British doctors isolated people who were worried, sad and anxious and predicted they'd be the ones to suffer heart attacks. Over a five-year period, a check of the subjects' health proved the doctors had been 67 percent accurate.

And at the Washington University School of Medicine in St. Louis, scientists using only a psychological test were 73 percent correct in choosing the undiagnosed cancer victims from a group of men with lung problems.

Fortunately, there's good news, too. First, it's also been shown that there is a positive relationship between good health and being satisfied, having friends and enjoying other pluses in your life. And you can make your life better in all of these areas.

Second, other studies have suggested that it's not hard times in themselves that make us vulnerable to disease. Instead, the trouble seems to come from the feeling of being trapped — what we humans feel as hopelessness and helplessness. The good news to be found in studies like these is that people can learn to improve their ability to cope and thus increase their happiness quotient.

Of course the question of what happiness *is*, exactly, has been bugging philosophers and great thinkers through the ages (see "The World's Great Thinkers on . . . Happiness" on pages 50-51). Many theorize that, as with our Seven Happiness Soup (see page 46), the ingredients vary according to individual taste, given a basically good stock.

MOST HAPPY WOMAN

The happiest person on the North American continent is a 40-year-old woman Unitarian minister who lives in Canada with her husband, who loves her just as much as she loves him. Of course, this person probably doesn't exist. Rather, she is a statistical creation who serves to demonstrate the absurdity of trying to fit yourself to a formula.

Her profile is a composite drawn from surveys and studies of more than 100,000 people done by psychologist Jonathan Freedman, Ph.D., and many others and discussed in his book *Happy People.* Clearly, you don't have to study divinity, be married or move to the far side of Niagara Falls to be happy. In fact, at least 60 percent of us do consider ourselves moderately happy. Our happiness is not necessarily tied to our income levels. (Grinding poverty *is* tied to unhappiness, though. A Gallup poll done in an underdeveloped country revealed satisfaction levels as low as 20 percent.)

The survey of 100,000 people also showed we are happy when we feel that life has meaning, whether we draw that from religion or some other source. We tend to be happier when we are in a loving relationship, when we have friends and when we are employed.

No one but you can tell if any of these things will make *you* happy, of course. But based on this survey and other well-conducted studies, and on interviews with psychologists and other experts, we have put together a list of suggestions—ideas you might want to try in your own pursuit of happiness.

Get a Job. People love to complain about their bosses and the workaday routine (maybe that's part of the fun). And we make hits of songs like "9 to 5" and "Take This Job and Shove It." But our terrible secret is that we love to work. Employed people are more satisfied than the idle. One recent University of Michigan study of 2,500 Americans revealed that we prefer working at our jobs to watching TV, going to the movies or reading books or newspapers.

Talk It Over. Some psychologists tell us that we often do not know what we feel until we start to talk about it. And talking—not just social chitchat, but the kind of talk that eases your soul when something is bothering you—is a very healthy thing to do, says James Pennebaker, Ph.D., who has supported this notion through a series of studies. His research shows that people who confide in each other live healthier lives.

"Many people visit their doctors just to get someone to listen to them," a magazine article once joked. But you can cut down the number of times you *need* to talk to your doctor by confiding in someone else.

Give Your Body a Boost. You can change your mood and your self-image with the simple life ingredients of food, sleep and exercise. The right kinds and amounts of each can make or break your enjoyment of your life.

Give to Live. Can unconditional love—love that gives without looking for a return, that is given for the sake of giving—be measured in a test tube? Not yet, but scientists are working on it.

They've found, for instance, that merely watching a movie about Mother Teresa, the Nobel prize-winning nun who lovingly cares for Calcutta's dying, helped college students fight off disease. Harvard professor of psychology David McClelland, Ph.D., who conducted the study, is convinced the results are connected with the students' "altruistic state of mind."

Years ago the famed psychiatrist and psychologist Alfred Adler claimed that any depression could be cured in seven days. All patients had to do was to think each day of something to do for another person that would make a significant difference to that person.

Most of us know instinctively that helping someone else makes us feel better. And no doubt that's why

Are You a Positive Person?

Whether you see the glass as half full or half empty can affect your health. Take our test to see how positive you are.

	1 Never	2 Rarely	3 Some-times	4 Usually	5 Always
1. When the unexpected forces you to change your plans, are you quick to spot a hidden advantage in this new situation?					
2. When you catch a stranger staring at you, do you conclude it's because he or she finds you attractive?					
3. Do you like most of the people you meet?					
4. When you think about next year, do you tend to think you'll be better off than you are now?					
5. Do you often stop to admire things of beauty?					
6. When someone finds fault with you or something you've done, can you tell the difference between useful criticism and "sour grapes," which is better off ignored?					
7. Do you praise your spouse/best friend/lover more often than you criticize him or her?					
8. Do you believe the human race will survive into the 21st century?					
9. Are you surprised when a friend lets you down?					
10. Do you think of yourself as happy?					
11. If a policeman stopped you for speeding when you were quite certain you weren't, would you firmly argue your case and even take it to court to prove you were right?					
12. Do you feel comfortable making yourself the butt of your own jokes?					
13. Do you believe that, overall, your state of mind has had a positive effect on your physical health?					
14. If you made a list of your 10 favorite people, would you be on it?					
15. When you think back over the past few months, do you tend to remember your little successes before your setbacks and failures?					

Scoring

If you scored 65 or over, consider yourself a "superstar"—someone whose optimism is a powerful, healing force.

60-65: Excellent—you're a genuine positive thinker.

55-60: Good—you're a positive thinker . . . sometimes.

50-55: Fair—your positive side and your negative side are about evenly matched.

50 and below: Do you see any consistent negative patterns? Where could you improve?

Seven Happiness Soup

Happiness is a warm bowl of soup. The Chinese think so, anyway. To them it's "the stomach warmer," and they won't start a meal without it. Here's a recipe for a classic Chinese soup that's a "double mouthful"—delicious *and* nutritious. You may substitute ingredients if you wish, but according to ancient wisdom, keep the number of vegetables at 7 for maximum happiness.

Makes 4 servings

2 shiitake mushrooms (each about 1½'' × 1½''), soaked and shredded
1 square (4'' × 4'') or 3 tablespoons threads wakame, soaked and shredded
½ cup bok choy, white only, cut into matchstick-size pieces
1 1''-long chunk daikon, cut into matchstick-size pieces
2 scallions, cut into matchstick-size pieces
1 medium carrot, cut into matchstick-size pieces

4 cups chicken stock
1 clove garlic
1 ⅛'' slice ginger root
2 tablespoons orange juice (or juice of 1 medium orange)
1 tablespoon rice vinegar
½ cup shredded spinach
1 teaspoon sesame oil

In a medium saucepan, combine mushrooms, wakame, bok choy, daikon, scallions, carrots, chicken stock, garlic, ginger, orange juice and vinegar. Simmer, stirring occasionally, for 15 minutes.

Add spinach and sesame oil and simmer for 5 minutes more.

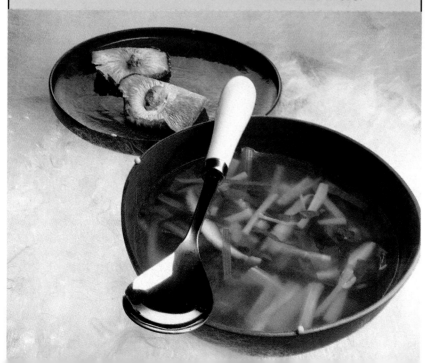

more than 50 percent of Americans contribute their time to some voluntary activity, whether it's helping an elderly neighbor, for example, or leading a Boy Scout troop, according to a recent Gallup poll.

Our motives don't have to be pure, say experts. There's nothing wrong with seeking an outlet for giving because we're lonely, bored or distressed—as long as the person we're helping wants to be helped.

Beverly DeFiore, a 31-year-old nurse, admits she joined Big Brothers-Big Sisters, an organization that matches children who need extra adult attention with adults who have time to give, because she "needed someone."

An injury that included two broken fingers and required her to wear a neck brace and a foot brace forced her to leave her job. She was devastated over having to quit. She felt like a failure.

Getting close to her "little sister," Aurora, "closer than I ever expected I could get," gave her a purpose. "I found out I wasn't all bad," says Beverly.

Whether it's shoveling snow off your neighbor's walk, visiting elderly residents of a nursing home or teaching an adult how to read, the act of reaching out your hand to help a fellow human being is likely to make you feel terrific. It's how Judy, the most cheerful worker in a small company, explains her good humor. "I love to do things for people. I love to do little extra things for people. There's no one in this building I wouldn't help."

Let the Fun Shine In. Don't listen to fun experts to learn how to have fun—just do it. That's the advice of fun expert Geoffrey Godbey, Ph.D., a professor of recreation and parks at Pennsylvania State University, who says that fun can only be allowed to happen; it can't be made to happen.

Dogs and children have a natural sense of fun, he says, which makes them excellent choices as playmates. (This is probably why talking to, playing with and caring for children are Americans' favorite activities, according to the University of Michigan study.)

And practical jokes can be fun,

too. Dr. Godbey is an occasional writer of letters to friends notifying them of "awards" they've won from certain dignified "institutions." Taking his lead, you might reward your children for cleaning their rooms by awarding them certificates from the National Trash Haulers Association, for example. But be sure your jokes are in good spirit, he cautions. Cruelty is never fun.

Dr. Godbey gives his good-old-fashioned-fun seal of approval to amusement parks, too. And you needn't be accompanied by children. Half of the visitors to theme parks like Six Flags over Texas who are over age 55 are there without children, Dr. Godbey's research shows.

Fun should be its own reward, he says. It should make you lose self-consciousness and lose track of time. Whether it's pinball or camel racing or watching the ants on the sidewalk, it shouldn't have to be good for you—just something you find pleasurable.

Perk Up Your Appearance. The old comic-strip solution to a woman's depression—buying a new hat—deserves more than a laugh. Improving your physical appearance—like your clothes, physique, hair or skin—can be a shortcut to improved self-confidence and self-esteem, says one psychologist. It actually is an instance where you *can* change the inside by changing the outside, say behavior experts.

Then learn to accept—and absorb, really letting them soak in—the compliments that follow. It's another way to feel better about yourself, experts say.

Relax. By learning a relaxation technique, you provide a good basis for all kinds of treatments and open yourself up to new influences.

Laugh. "The arrival of a good clown exercises a more beneficial influence upon the health of a town than 20 asses laden with drugs," said a famous physician a few centuries ago. And modern medicine is starting to catch up with him. Some hospitals now have "humor rooms," for instance (see "Medicinal Laughter" on page 94).

How to Build Trust in Friendship

Friends you can trust are a tremendous boon to your health, research shows. To build trusting friendships you must learn "to deal honestly and directly with your feelings about the relationship," says Lillian Rubin, Ph.D., author of *Just Friends*. And it's the difficult feelings—the ones you fear may hurt your friend or make you too vulnerable—that you must work hardest to express, she says.

It's not a matter of blurting out every thought that crosses your mind, cautions Dr. Rubin, but of communicating important thoughts and feelings. She cites as an example the unhappiness felt by one of her patients, whose imagination went wild when a friend became distant.

What had happened, says Dr. Rubin, was that the friend had become uncomfortable with the patient's desire for a rigidly structured relationship—phone calls every Monday and dinner every Tuesday. Rather than say this, she'd backed away.

"If something is interfering with a friendship, you must express it," says Dr. Rubin. "You'll hurt your friend much more by suddenly shifting ground with no explanation. This kind of unexplained action leads to paranoia—the opposite of trust."

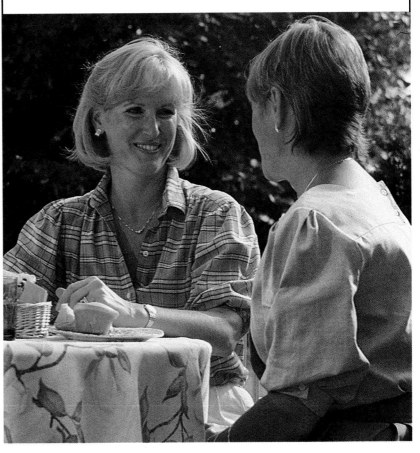

But more than getting you well, humor can *keep* you healthy. Humor keeps your frame of mind bright as it punctures pomposity and redresses injustice. It sees you through rough times. It releases tension. It's probably the most constructive way of handling anger. "It is the truth which is rarely spoken," says Harold Greenwald, Ph.D., a psychologist and author of *The Happy Person*, who says his patients sometimes ask him, "Are you the real Dr. Greenwald? Or are you some nut who's tied him up and thrown him in the closet?"

You can decide to develop your sense of humor simply by exposing yourself to things that make you laugh and by beginning to look for life's little quirks and the opportunities to point them out.

Lighten Up. A noted anthropology professor dances the can-can for his classes to demonstrate bipedality. Yale professor and cancer surgeon Bernard Siegal, M.D., plays country music in the operating room. One New England psychologist invented a foam-padded alarm clock that can be turned off only by being hurled against a wall. And Donald Duck comic books are being taught as serious literature at Vanderbilt University. Does it all seem a little, well, silly? Being playful won't make you into a superficial person, says Dr. Greenwald. Like one accomplished physics professor, you might consider decorating your mirror with a sign: "This person is not to be taken too seriously."

Of course, to say to someone who has serious emotional wounds that they shouldn't take themselves so seriously "is an insult," cautions psychologist Laidily MacBride. "Their pain *must* be taken seriously before they can possibly enjoy anything. Their trust in goodness must be restored."

Turn Negatives into Positives. When you look at your lawn, do you see the four-leaf clovers or the dandelions? And do you see the dandelions as weeds or as pretty yellow flowers? Could you manage to see them as a golden opportunity, and weeding as a chance to get some sun, fresh air and a little exercise?

As our dandelion example shows, if you see a problem as an opportunity—perhaps an opportunity to learn and grow when the situation is painful—it isn't a problem anymore.

This principle can be applied in almost any situation, because every negative does have a positive side. For example, when one psychologist's teenage son recently backed a pickup truck into her car, causing $1,375 worth of damage which the insurance company refused to pay, she could have been angry and unhappy about her ruined finances. Instead, she reflected that "the beach is free and making love is free. Reading or playing with the baby's toes doesn't cost $1,375." She also saw it as an opportunity to learn—to scrutinize insurance policies before buying them.

Touch. If babies aren't held and fondled, they don't grow properly. They may even die. Grownups need friendly touching, too. But if we weren't brought up in households where physical reassurances were commonplace, we'll need training in Basic Hugging.

Practice, practice, practice, says family counselor Helen Colton, author of *The Gift of Touch.* You can

---

The Biology of Laughter

It can happen to you first as early as the age of 5 weeks. With luck, it should continue to occur perhaps 15 times a day for the rest of your life.

What takes place is a tightening of facial muscles that pulls the corners of your mouth up and to the sides. Your eyes brighten as tear glands produce moisture. Your heart beats faster and your muscles contract spasmodically. You breathe in deeply as your diaphragm's movement massages your internal organs. After it's over, muscle tension eases and your heart assumes a more relaxed pace than before the episode began.

You have undergone a complex physiological response involving several biochemical, hormonal and circulatory happenings. In short, you have laughed.

hug family, friends, co-workers, even bosses. And slowly you can advance from the common A-frame hug, where touching is done only at shoulder level, to a truer, warmer hug.

Know and Like Yourself. We all have a "hanging judge" inside, says Dr. Greenwald. Often the voice of an overactive conscience or an unrealistic set of expectations, this judge tells us our performance is never quite good enough. That negative voice must be controlled if we are to be happy, he says.

How? First, you must learn to recognize the hanging judge's voice and ask yourself questions. If you want to put off doing the dishes until morning, does that really make you a bad person? Or is it more important to spend the time right now with your family?

One woman finds it useful to remember the phrase, "When I'm hurting, I look to see if the whip is in my hand." Too often, says Dr. Greenwald, we are harder on ourselves than we would ever be on someone else.

Act As If. An effective way to change behavior and attitudes, says Dr. Greenwald, is the simple expedient of "acting as if." If you want to lose weight, for instance, act as if you had already lost it. If you eat like a thin person, you will become thin.

This technique works on more complex levels, too, Dr. Greenwald says. If you want to be more cheerful, for example, think how you'd behave if you were more cheerful, then act that way. You'll become more cheerful. Want to be less afraid? Act as if you are unafraid, and soon you will feel that way.

Even arranging your face to reflect how you'd like to feel can help you feel that way, says a scientist who has demonstrated that facial expressions produce characteristic patterns in the nervous system.

Live in Today. Don't worry about the mistakes of the past or the problems of the future. Ask yourself, "What can I do about it right now?" If there is something, do it. If not, move on.

Cry. A suggestion that you cry in a chapter on happiness? Yes. Experts say that it's an excellent way to ease tension and release your feelings. There's speculation, too, that tears of sadness may carry off chemicals that contribute to your blue feelings.

Decide to Be Happy. "When you don't have problems, you're dead," notes Dr. Greenwald. "But just to make up your mind to be a happy person is a tremendous contribution to the world. It takes courage to be happy. Remember that this is it. This is not a dress rehearsal."

Henny Youngman's Best One-Liners

My wife is a light eater—as soon as it's light she starts eating.

My doctor is an eye, ear, nose, throat and wallet specialist!

My mother was 88 years old and she never used glasses—she drank right out of the bottle!

"How is your wife?"
"Compared to who?"

There's nothing wrong with our foreign policy that faith, hope and clarity couldn't cure!

Am I forgetful? Last night I forgot the Alamo!

When entering a restaurant, I say to the manager, "Give me a table near a waiter, please."

He plays like Paderewski—he uses both hands.

Indian girl marries Jewish boy. They have to give their new son a name to please both sides of the family. They name him "Whitefish."

Here it is election time, and once again isn't it amazing how many wide open spaces there are—entirely surrounded by teeth.

I miss my wife's cooking—as often as I can.

It's a bad day when you hear on the airplane intercom, "This is your captain speaking; they will never take me alive."

The World's Great _____
Thinkers on . . .

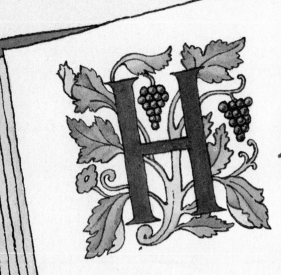

HAPPINESS

Be content with your lot; one cannot be first in everything.
— *Aesop*

Happiness is activity.
— *Aristotle*

Indeed, man wishes to be happy even when he so lives as to make happiness impossible.
— *St. Augustine*

The game isn't over till it's over.
— *Yogi Berra*

The bird of paradise alights only upon the hand that does not grasp.
— *John Berry*

He that is of a merry heart hath a continual feast.
— *Proverbs 15:15*

A merry heart doeth good like a medicine.
— *Proverbs 17:22*

Happiness, *n.* An agreeable sensation arising from contemplating the misery of another.
— *Ambrose Bierce*

The Angel that presided o'er my birth
Said, "Little creature, formed of joy and mirth,
Go love without the help of any thing on earth."
— *William Blake*

All who joy would win
Must share it—Happiness was born a Twin.
— *Lord Byron*

How many cares one loses wh[en] one decides not to be someth[ing] but to be someone.
— *Coco Ch[anel]*

"The prince keeps [a] torto[ise] carefully enclosed in a ch[est in] his ancestral temple. Now [would] this tortoise rather be d[ead to] have its remains venera[ted, or] would it rather be alive [and] wagging its tail in the [mud?]"
"It would rather [be alive] and wagging its tail [in the] mud."
"Begone!" cried Ch[uang:] "too will wag my ta[il in the] mud."

Those pleasures [are] physical.

With coarse [rice to eat,] water to drin[k, and my] arm for a pil[low, I have] joy in the m[idst of these.] Riches and [honors acquired by] unrighteo[usness are to me as a] floating c[loud.]

Illusory [happiness is better] than ge[nuine misery.]

Happ[iness is not] happ[iness unless shared with] me[n.]

...he hour, and leave no ...for a repentance or an ...al—that is happiness.
— *Ralph Waldo Emerson*

...he chiefest point of happi- ...that a man is willing to be ...he is.
— *Erasmus*

...man felicity is produced not ...much by great pieces of good ...tune that seldom happen as ...little advantages that occur ...very day.
— *Benjamin Franklin*

A great obstacle to happiness is to anticipate too great a happiness.
— *Fontenelle*

Modern man's happiness consists in the thrill of looking at the shop windows and in buying all that he can afford to buy either for cash or on installments.
— *Erich Fromm*

Your joy is your sorrow unmasked. And the selfsame well from which your laughter rises was oftentimes filled with your tears.
— *Kahlil Gibran*

He is the happiest man who can connect the end of his life with its beginning.
— *Goethe*

[Happiness] always looks small while you hold it in your hands, but let it go, and you learn at once how big and precious it is.
— *Maxim Gorky*

Illusory joy is often worth more than genuine sorrow.
— *René Descartes*

The search for happiness is one of the chief sources of unhappiness.
— *Eric Hoffer*

Happiness is like coke— something you get as a byproduct in the process of making something else.
— *Aldous Huxley*

You do not need to leave your room. Remain sitting at your table and listen. Do not even listen, simply wait. Do not even wait, be quite still and solitary. The world will freely offer itself to you to be unmasked, it has no choice, it will roll in ecstasy at your feet.
— *Franz Kafka*

No matter how dull, or how mean, or how wise a man is, he feels that happiness is his indisputable right.
— *Helen Keller*

Success is getting what you want; happiness is wanting what you get.
— *Charles F. Kettering*

If an Arab in the desert were suddenly to discover a spring in his tent, and so would always be able to have water in abundance, how fortunate he would consider himself—so too, when a man, who as a physical being is always turned toward the outside, thinking that his happiness lies outside him, finally turns inward and discovers that the source is within him; not to mention his discovery that the source is his relation to Good.
— *Sören Kierkegaard*

Happiness does not lie in happiness, but in the achievement of it.
— *Fyodor Dostoevsky*

Happiness is in the taste, and not in the things.
— *La Rochefoucauld*

I get by with a little help from my friends. Let it be.
— *John Lennon and Paul McCartney*

Ask yourself whether you are happy, and you cease to be so.
— *John Stuart Mill*

Happy are the people whose annals are tiresome.
— *Montesquieu*

Most people ask for happiness on condition. Happiness can only be felt if you don't see any condition.
— *Arthur Rubinstein*

The greatest happiness you can have is knowing that you do not necessarily require happiness.
— *William Saroyan*

Pain is short, and joy is eternal.
— *Schiller*

Happiness is a warm puppy.
— *Charles Schulz*

A merry heart goes all the day, Your sad tires in a mile-a.
— *William Shakespeare*

Man is meant for happiness and this happiness is in him, in the satisfaction of the daily needs of his existence.
— *Leo Tolstoy*

The most beautiful thing we can experience is the mysterious. It is the source of all true art and science.
— *Albert Einstein*

5

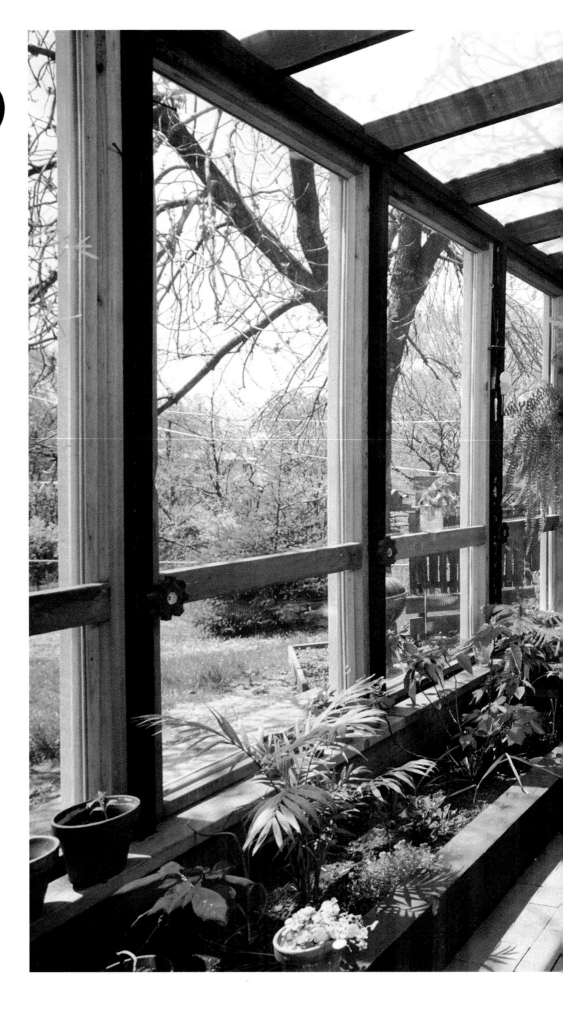

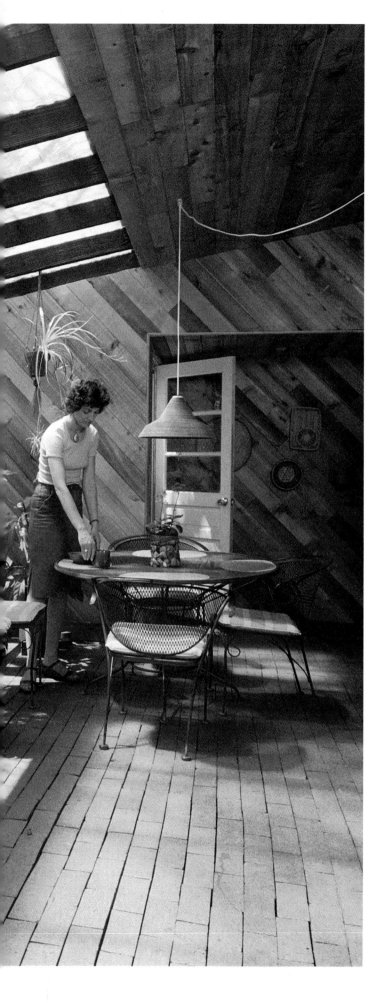

Mastering Your Personal Environment

Maybe you can't stop the acid rain, but you can control your home environment.

L ook around your living room. Who decorated it? Who decided that an Oriental rug was nicer than wall-to-wall or that family photos were better than paintings? Who picked out the shades, the drapes, the curtains?

Now close your eyes and listen. What do you hear? Kids playing baseball?

And sniff. Is that lemon verbena in the garden? Who planted it? Who figured out that the same breeze that's pushing back the curtains would carry the scent through the window and under your nose?

The odds are ten to one that you did. You decided what made the room feel right, what made it feel like home. Oh, sure, you may have to share some of the decision-making with your spouse or your kids. But you are in charge of the space in which you play or eat or sleep or just plain vegetate. You also can help shape the environment of your workplace, although to a lesser degree. Even if you're standing on an assembly line in Toronto, you can shove a rubber mat under your feet and headphones of one sort or another over your ears.

And it's important that you do. Whether at home or at work, your environment is an extension of yourself, an external womb intended to shelter, stimulate and nourish. If you can make it clean, quiet, healthy and safe, you'll flourish. And here's the way to do it.

Just how safe is your home? Let's take a tour and find out. Go out the front entrance, turn

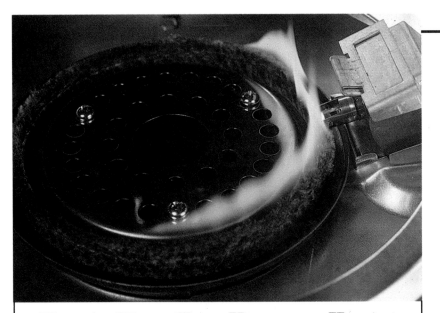

How to Clean Your Kerosene Heater

In one recent year, nearly 700 people died and 4,000 people were injured from burns, fires and carbon monoxide poisoning caused by the use of supplemental heaters, reports the Consumer Product Safety Commission. And one reason was improper maintenance. The National Kerosene Heater Association recommends that before using your heater in the fall, reread your instruction manual and closely follow the manual's cleaning instructions. Rinse the empty kerosene tank with small amounts of pure, clear (1K) kerosene only, then check the wick and replace it if necessary. In the fall and throughout the season, clean the heater thoroughly, wiping dust and soot from the heater cabinet, wick and working parts. Replace batteries as needed, check operation of the igniter, and regularly test the shut-off device. Once the unit is clean, refuel it, then allow the wick 30 to 60 minutes to absorb the fuel. Ignite the unit and check that it's operating properly.

around and face the door. Are there any stairs or steps?

If there are, do you have a handrail that runs all the way from top step to bottom step and doesn't stop short at either end? Safety experts at Johns Hopkins School of Public Health suggest that you do. They also suggest that stair edges be prominently marked, covered with a nonskid tread and well lit.

So how do your stairs measure up? Give yourself an "A" if your stairs are already safe. Clearly, you won't be one of the over

770,000 people each year who fall down the stairs—and land in the emergency room.

MAKE YOUR BEDROOM SAFE

Now let's go inside and zero in on the most dangerous room in the home: the bedroom. For each of the four most frequent kinds of fatal accidents occurring inside the home— falls, fire, poisoning and suffocation—the place they're most likely to happen is the bedroom, says the National Safety Council (NSC).

Fortunately, the bedroom is easily made safe. Just look around. Are there any small rugs in the room? If there are, check to see that they have a nonskid backing. Apply double-sided tape or foam rubber if they don't and tack down or repair any loose or frayed edges.

Are there medications in your bedroom? Many of us need to take medication through the night, so we leave it beside the bed. In that case, safety experts suggest we leave only enough on the bedside table for a single dose or a single night. And always turn on the light so you can see what you're taking, they advise.

Is there an ashtray beside the bed? Maybe you should think about moving it away from the bed and closer to a chair. People who fall asleep while smoking in bed cause thousands of fires and fire-related deaths.

Now look out into the hall. Do you have a smoke detector mounted there on the ceiling right outside the bedroom? If not, you should think about installing one (see "Where to Put Smoke Detectors"). Smoke detectors save lives. The best ones cost less than $40 and many are available for under $20.

MAKE YOUR BATHROOM SAFE

Now let's take a stroll down the hall and into the bathroom, where more than 200,000 people are estimated to be injured annually, according to the NSC. The most common injury occurs when you slip getting out of a tub or shower. Worse, about 200 people drown every year, many of whom probably fall and knock themselves out. And it's doubly tragic because most of these accidents are easily prevented by using a suction-type rubber mat or safety strips in the bottom of your tub or shower.

You might want to check out bathtubs with a permanent slip-resistant bottom when you remodel or move. Other safety features you also might want to consider then include recessed faucets and soap dishes; fixtures made of softer materials than the standard ceramic, such as fiberglass; and grab bars that can be firmly anchored into the wall studs.

MAKE YOUR KITCHEN SAFE

Now let's take a look at your kitchen. What, for example, do you keep in your kitchen cupboards? Are dangerous items like ammonia, oven cleaner and drain openers safely locked up? How about your other cleaning supplies, liquor and medicines? They, too, should be stored where no one can get into them by mistake or by curious intent.

As for the rest of your kitchen, make sure your stove, refrigerator, dishwasher and other major electrical applicances are grounded. If you're not sure, you may want to call an electrician to check. And while he or she is there, you may want to ask about adding ground-fault circuit interrupters (GFCI) to your kitchen outlets, if you don't already have them.

The GFCIs, which look like switchplates with a test and reset button in the middle, will prevent electric shock from faulty equipment by monitoring and interrupting the flow of electricity. If you touch the GFCI-protected switch of a garbage disposal with wet hands, for example, the GFCI will shut off the electricity so you don't get any more than the initial zap. In other words, your life may have been saved by a little gadget that costs less than $20 to $30 if installed by a professional.

THE YARD, TOO

Now let's take a look outside. Whether you have a 10-foot-square cement

Where to Put Smoke Detectors

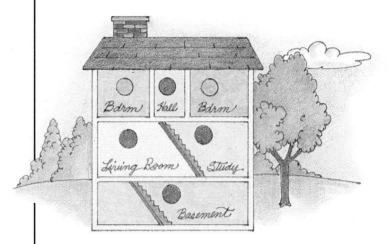

Smoke detectors save lives. Their piercing horns get you out of bed and out of the house before fires get you trapped. Three types are available: the ionization detector, which is most sensitive to rapidly burning fires; the photoelectric detector, which senses slow-burning, smoldering fires; and the combination detector, which includes both types. But whichever type you buy, the National Fire Protection Association suggests you install them in the immediate vicinity of the bedrooms and on each level of the home where there are no bedrooms—including the basement.

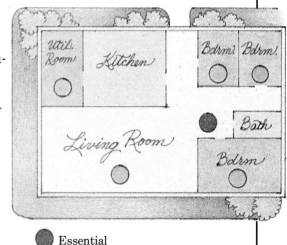

● Essential
●+○ Ideal

courtyard outside a rented apartment, a 10-acre testament to the skill of your gardeners or something in between, the outside of your home should be as safe and comfortable as the inside. So look around and see if there are any obvious hazards.

Are trees trimmed, for example, so that no dead or broken branches or limbs can fall on people or power lines? Are hedges and shrubs clipped so they don't obscure the presence of a child moving toward a parking lot, street or driveway?

Are electrical tools grounded

Water Treatment Methods

	Hardness	Trace metals	Odor	THMs	Hydrogen sulfide	Iron	Nitrates	Bacteria
Reverse osmosis	●	●	●			●	●	●
Ion exchange	●¹					●²	●³	
Distillation	●	●	●		●	●	●	●
Chlorination			●		●	●		●
Activated carbon filtration			●	●				
Manganese green-sand filtration					●⁴	●⁴		

¹cation resin ³anion resin
²with hardness and ferrous iron limits ⁴regenerated with potassium permanganate

Not all water-treatment methods are created equal. Each one is designed to remove specific substances from your water. Have your water tested, then consult the chart above to see which water treatment method is right for you. Keep in mind that more than one system may be necessary to assure pure, healthful water. Cheers!

and used only with heavy-duty outdoor extension cords? Are swimming pools fenced in and covered or drained when not in use? Are garage door controls out of a child's reach?

And how about your walks, steps and porches? Are they in good repair and clear of debris?

Approximately 25 percent of all accidental home injuries and deaths occur outside in a yard or garage, on a porch or steps. But remember the old saying, "There's no such thing as an accident." With just a little care and forethought, there's not one reason why anything should happen to *you*.

MAKE YOUR HOME FIRE RESISTANT

But how can you protect yourself from fire?

Your best defense is prevention. And prevention, fire experts say, means cleaning the grease off kitchen exhaust fans; regularly vacuuming workshop sawdust; tightly sealing all cans of paint, paint thinner, rubber cement and other flammable liquids; discarding oily rags outdoors after use; not overloading outlets; replacing frayed wires; and avoiding the accumulation of piles of flammable materials such as magazines and newspapers.

But fire prevention also means that you should pay careful attention to any heat sources in your home. Keep auxiliary heating devices away from curtains, bedding and upholstery. Cover fireplaces with a screen to prevent sparks from flying out onto rugs and furniture. If you burn artificial logs, read the instructions on the log's wrapper and follow them exactly. And when you clean your fireplace and throw out the ashes, make sure they're cold.

But fire safety is more than just prevention. It's also preparation. What, for example, would your family do if a fire started at night while you were asleep?

Your first line of defense is comprised of properly installed and maintained smoke detectors. A study in Montgomery County, Maryland, indicates that fire deaths in the county were cut in half after a law requiring smoke detectors went into effect.

Next, you need practice. Here's the script.

Time: Late at night.

Place: The hallway just outside your bedroom. Pretend that tendrils of smoke are beginning to drift through the corridor. Without warning, the earsplitting horn of a smoke detector pierces the night. An emergency light, triggered by the alarm, flashes through the smoke to illuminate the hall.

Action: This is a drill, but you act as though it is real. You and your family leap out of bed. You do not stop to look for your shoes, your jewelry, your pants or your pets. You move quickly toward an outside door, dropping to your belly and crawling under the smoke where necessary. When you get near the door, you find that it is blocked by flames, but no one panics. (Since you run through this little play four times a year, pretending the fire is in a different location each time, you all know what to do.) You turn and head for the bedroom in which a portable fire escape is kept under the bed. When you're all in the room, you close the bedroom door, then open the window. Your spouse shoves the lightweight ladder over the sill and attaches it exactly the way the ladder's instruction booklet advises, then it's over and down for each of you.

FIGHT FIRE WITH—WHAT?

If a fire is small, however, some people try to control it before putting the escape plan into action. In this case, safety experts suggest you keep a fire extinguisher in the kitchen and basement.

But be careful what kind you buy. Each type of extinguisher is designed for a different type of fire. Ordinary paper and wood fires, which firefighters call Class A, require water, dry chemical or foam extinguishers. Class B fires, which include flammable or combustible liquids such as greases or paint solvents and thinners, need dry chemical, carbon dioxide or foam extinguishers. Class C fires, involving electrical equipment and wires, call for dry chemical or carbon dioxide extinguishers.

To simplify matters, most fire safety experts suggest you buy a *multipurpose* dry chemical extinguisher. You can identify it by the "A:B:C" code on the label, which indicates that the extinguisher is approved for all three types of fires.

When you remodel or build a new home, however, you may want to look into more modern—and more efficient—ways to fight a fire. You may in particular want to add a built-in sprinkler system. As Gary Hilbert, a researcher with the International Association of Fire Chiefs, points out, no one has yet died in a home or business with a properly installed and maintained sprinkler system.

MAKE IT HEALTHY

But making your home safe from fire and accidental injury is only a part of creating a nourishing, supportive environment. Just as important is making your home healthy.

Fortunately, in some cases the task may very well be as easy as opening a window, because a major source of unhealthfulness in our homes is indoor air pollution. And some of the major pollutants are tobacco smoke, formaldehyde, carbon monoxide and radon (see "Indoor Air Pollution" on page 58).

Years ago, most of us weren't as likely to be affected by these substances when—in our unenlightened energy unconsciousness—our homes were uncaulked, unweatherstripped, uninsulated, single-paned and generally drafty.

Spider Plants Clean the Air

Spider plants may become standard fixtures on future space flights if the scientists at NASA's National Space Technology Lab have anything to say about it. The scientists, who have been looking for a way to purify the air in spacecrafts, have discovered that spider plants—and others, too—efficiently remove formaldehyde. Can we use this "high-tech" info? Sure. It's possible that 8 to 15 plants can clean the formaldehyde from an average home's air.

Indoor Air Pollution

Pollutant	Description	Possible Health Effects	Sources in Homes	Ways to Reduce Exposure
Asbestos	Fibrous material.	Lung and stomach cancer, mesothelioma, fibrotic lung diseases.	Any older construction material used for fireproofing, insulating or spackling.	• Stay away from it.
Benzo-(a)-pyrene (BaP)	A tarry organic particle from incomplete combustion.	Nose, throat and eye irritation, lung cancer, emphysema, heart disease, bronchitis, respiratory infections.	Tobacco smoke, wood smoke.	• Avoid smoking tobacco inside. • Be sure pipe from wood stove does not leak. • Vent combustion appliances outdoors. • Change air filters regularly. • Increase ventilation.
Carbon monoxide	Colorless, odorless, tasteless gas from all fuel burning.	Lung ailments. Impaired vision and brain functioning. Fatal in very high concentrations.	Kerosene heaters, wood stoves, attached garages, tobacco smoke, unvented gas stoves.	• Be sure gas stoves are properly vented. • Install exhaust fans above gas stoves. • Keep gas appliances properly adjusted.
Formaldehyde	Strong-smelling, colorless gas, a component of some insulation and of glues used in making plywood, particle board and textiles.	Nose, throat and eye irritation, possibly nasal cancer or brain cancer. Short-term memory loss, increased anxiety and slight changes in adaptation to darkness.	Various materials, including urea-formaldehyde foam insulation (UFFI), particle board, plywood, furniture, drapes and carpet, shampoo. Also in tobacco smoke.	• Use materials that are relatively low in formaldehyde. Examples are low-formaldehyde particle board and exterior-grade plywood, which release less formaldehyde than interior grades. • Open windows or install air-to-air heat exchanger.
Household chemicals	Organic compounds found in household products.	Irritation of skin, eyes, nose and throat, effects on central nervous system and metabolic processes.	Synthetic materials, pesticides, aerosol sprays, cleaning agents, paints.	• Follow label directions for use. • Use chemicals only in well-ventilated areas. • Store chemicals in a garage or outdoor shed.
Nitrogen oxides	Colorless, tasteless gas formed during combustion.	Lung damage. Lung disease after long exposure.	Kerosene heaters, unvented gas stoves.	• Install exhaust fans above gas stoves. • Keep gas appliances properly adjusted. • Increase ventilation.
Radon	Odorless, colorless radioactive gas, a decay product of uranium, which occurs naturally in the earth's crust.	Believed responsible for about 5 percent of all lung cancers; 24 percent of all lung cancers in nonsmokers.	Earth and rock beneath home. Building materials such as concrete, brick, stone or drywall made of phosphogypsum. Water.	• Increase ventilation. • Use exhaust fans while running water. • Add crawlspace vents. • Avoid home-tightening measures like weatherstripping. • Install air-to-air heat exchanger. • Seal cracks and other openings in basement floor. • Double-coat foundation with specially prepared epoxy or oil emulsion paints.

Today, however, many of us have sealed our homes to keep in the warmed air of winter, the cooled air of summer and a few of our hard-earned energy dollars as well.

But we've also sealed in the pollutants. That's why simply opening a window can sometimes make our home more healthful. It can let out the carbon monoxide generated by our gas-fired heaters and the formaldehyde that can "outgas" from the glues or adhesives in the plywood or particle-board components of our furniture and from synthetic carpeting. It can even reduce the level of radon, a gas believed to be the second leading cause of lung cancer. The gas, which is both odorless and colorless, is given off during the decay process of uranium, a radioactive ore found in almost all soil and rocks.

THE "HOTTEST" LITTLE HOUSE IN THE WORLD

Admittedly, it did take a little more than open windows to get rid of the radon in the home of Diane Watras, a 33-year-old Pennsylvania homemaker and mother of two. Diane and her husband, Stan, have the honor of owning the "hottest" little house in the world. And "hot" has nothing to do with temperature. It has to do with radioactivity. Their split-level home had been built directly on top of a rock. What they didn't know then was that the rock contained low-grade uranium. In places, the rock was directly below the basement and family room, and the radon gas emitted by its uranium pushed into the house through small cracks, as well as through construction joints and a basement drain.

Fortunately, says Diane, "We hadn't finished the family room." Otherwise, she notes, her two small sons, then aged 15 months and 3½ years, would have been using the area for play. As it was, she says, scientists told her that the family would be about six times more likely to develop lung cancer if they remained in their home.

When Diane and Stan received a letter from the Pennsylvania Department of Environmental Resources (DER) suggesting they find "a safer shelter," even such a hard decision as moving was made in a hurry. The family packed up and left the next day.

They were safe, but what was to be done about the house? Even though scientists could measure the radon and knew it was getting in, they didn't know where it was coming from or how the house might be fixed.

It was at that point that Philadelphia Electric Company (PE), stepped in and offered to fund a research project that would figure out how to get rid of the radon.

PE had initially been involved because Stan, an engineer at its Limerick nuclear power plant, had set off radiation alarms intended to warn workers of dangerous radiation levels within the plant. Stan, however, set them off as he arrived, not after he'd been on the job.

Given that information, it hadn't taken officials long to trace the radioactivity back to Stan's house. The big utility put Ed Kohler, one of its research engineers, in charge of the project to fix Stan's house, hired ARIX, a Colorado-based firm of architects, engineers and planners to come up with a remedial plan, and contracted Ronald F. Simon Construction, a local Pennsylvania builder, to carry it out.

MAKING IT RADON PROOF

Constantly monitoring radiation levels, the team of engineers, physicists and construction workers first dug a trench along the foundation walls of the Watras house. Then they installed a pipe to drain radon-polluted groundwater away from the house. Next, they lined the walls with Trocal, a 24-millimeter plastic sheet that—unlike conventional plastic such as polyethylene—could stop the passage of radon. That reduced the radon levels, but not enough for the family to move back in.

Next the team sealed all the cracks and construction joints in the basement, along with the basement drain. The radon levels dropped even more.

The team then applied a spe-

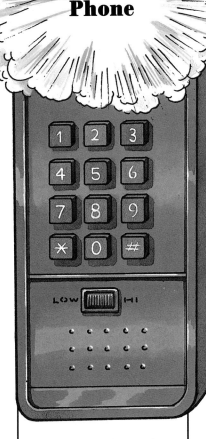

Blast-a-Phone

One blast from the ring of a cordless telephone directly into your ear can permanently destroy the tiny hair cells in the cochlea, says Jerome Goldstein, M.D., of the American Academy of Otolaryngology. The result can be permanent hearing loss, or even deafness. Next time a call comes in on your cordless, remember to flip off the ringer switch before you pick it up. You might even tape a reminder to the phone until turning it off becomes a habit.

Cigarettes: The Ingredients Label Would Read . . .

Think you're safe from lung cancer and other associated diseases because you don't smoke? Think again. A study of almost 8,000 adults in France indicated that nonsmoking husbands married to smoking wives lost 16 percent of their lung capacity. Nonsmoking wives married to smoking husbands lost 6 percent. That's because, standing next to Joe Blow, you inhale smoke coming from the burning tip of the cigarette, smoke that contains higher concentrations of many toxic and cancer-causing chemicals than the smoker himself inhales.

Here are some of the things you're breathing:

Acetone	Toxic	Nickel	Probable cause of cancer
Acetonitrile	Toxic		
Acrylonitrile	Known to cause cancer	Nicotine	Toxic
		Nitrogen oxides	Toxic
4-aminobiphenyl	Known to cause cancer	N-nitro- soanatabine	Suspected cause of cancers or tumors
Ammonia	Toxic	N-nitrosodie- thanolamine	Suspected cause of cancers or tumors
Aniline	Toxic		
Arsenic	Known to cause cancer	N-nitrosodie- thylamine	Suspected cause of cancers or tumors
Benzene	Known to cause cancer		
Benzo-(a)-pyrene	Probable cause of cancer	N-nitrosodi- methyl- amine	Probable cause of cancer
Cadmium	Probable cause of cancer	N-nitrosopyr- rolidine	Suspected cause of cancers or tumors
Carbon dioxide	Toxic		
Carbon monoxide	Toxic	O-toluidine	Suspected cause of cancers or tumors
Formaldehyde	Probable cause of cancer		
Hydrazine	Probable cause of cancer	Phenanthrene	Toxic
Hydrogen cyanide	Toxic	Polonium 210	Suspected cause of cancers or tumors
Methylquinoline	Toxic		
Naphthalene	Suspected cause of cancers or tumors	Pyridine	Toxic
		Quinoline	Toxic
1-naphthylamine	Suspected cause of cancers or tumors	Stigmasterol	Toxic
		Toluene	Toxic
		Vinyl chloride	Known to cause cancer
2-naphthylamine	Known to cause cancer	3-vinylpyridine	Toxic

The builder tore out the basement slab. And there was the rock, loaded with low-grade uranium.

Simon's crew used jackhammers to remove the top 10 inches of rock. Then they put pipes around the inside of the foundation to collect and vent radon seeping up from the rock. Next they covered the pipes and the rock with washed stone. Then they laid 30-pound felt over the stone, added Trocal and poured 2 inches of sand over the plastic to protect it. They finished the floor by pouring 4 inches of steel-reinforced concrete. The readings, says Ed Kohler, were finally low enough so that Stan, Diane and the kids could come home.

MAKE YOUR WATER CLEAN

But while you're cleaning up your air, maybe you should think about cleaning up your water, as well. Those of us with publicly supplied water may feel this job already has been done. However, we too may need extra help.

That's because the major source of pollution affecting those of us who use public water is chlorine, a disinfectant added to water to kill bacteria and viruses. Chlorination protects us from infectious hepatitis, poliomyelitis, cholera, typhoid fever, dysentery and a host of other intestinal infections.

The problem is that, while saving our lives, chlorine can also combine with the algae and other natural debris to form trihalomethanes (THMs), substances which have been strongly implicated in increasing the risk of various types of cancer—particularly cancer of the bladder.

Fortunately, THMs can be removed from our water, says Lucius Cole, technical director of the national Water Quality Association. There are three types of activated carbon filtration systems that will do the job, adds Cole—faucet-mounted devices that cost around $25, countertop models that run somewhere between $80 and $90, and under-sink systems that can cost up to $250.

All systems should have their filters changed periodically—twice as often as package inserts suggest, advises Cole—and each filter should be flushed of bacteria before you

cially prepared epoxy to other hard-to-reach parts of the foundation wall and installed perforated pipe along the top of that wall, with a smokestack-type vent running up through the house and out of the roof. Radon levels dropped, but almost before the team had time to celebrate, they jumped back up.

What was going on?

drink the water. To do that, let the water run between 15 and 45 seconds before you fill your cup, he suggests.

And—as always—you get what you pay for. Most of the small, single-faucet devices were designed for taste and odor control, reports Frank Bell, senior environmental engineer at the Environmental Protection Agency (EPA). The faucet-mounted units never removed more than 69 percent of the THMs encountered in EPA-sponsored tests, for example, while some of the larger, under-sink models removed up to 99 percent.

Moreover, the larger, under-sink systems can also remove at least some of the unsolicited chemicals that have come to haunt our daily lives. The pesticides Chlordane and DDT, as well as PCBs, can be removed by activated carbon filtration.

PRIVATE WELLS NEED HELP

But what of those of us who get our water from private wells rather than public systems?

Usually, the only thing we know for sure about our water is that it's not chlorinated. To find out what it does contain requires testing by a certified lab, which your local public health department can recommend.

Basic tests for bacteriological contamination, "hardness" and maybe one or two other items should cost less than $50. If you hear about local environmental problems—perhaps a landfill leaking its contents into the ground—you might want to have your water tested for those particular substances as well. (Of course, the cost jumps every time you add another item to the test list.)

By and large the major problem that individual well owners find is bacteriological, Bell says. In one study sponsored by the Virginia Department of Health, for example, 58 percent of the individual wells sampled were contaminated with coliform bacteria, organisms that frequently indicate the presence of more serious bacteria such as typhoid.

But remember what kills bacteria?

Right—chlorine. So if bacterial contamination turns out to be your

problem, says Cole, you should have a pump installed that will inject measured amounts of chlorine into your water system as it enters your home.

But what about chlorine's unwanted by-products, THMs? By adding chlorine, aren't you solving one problem by creating another?

Not quite. It's unlikely that chlorine could combine with algae or other types of naturally occurring materials to form THMs because that sort of organic debris should not be able to get into a properly constructed well. If you're concerned, however, you may want to have your local health department check the well.

ALL THE OTHER STUFF

Fortunately, most of the other water problems you're likely to encounter are cosmetic. Extra iron in the water, for example, is unsightly when it combines with oxygen at the top of your toilet bowl or in your washing machine. The rusty-red stains it leaves behind on the bowl and on clothes are nearly impossible to remove, and the chlorine bleach many people use to try to get rid of the stains actually makes them worse.

Fortunately, iron can be removed from your water by any one of five water-treatment systems—all of which cost less than the new wardrobe you'll need if the iron in your wash-water continues to rust-out your clothes. The systems (see "Water Treatment Methods" on page 56) include:

- Reverse osmosis, a system in which a separate cellophanelike membrane reduces not only iron but bacteria, trace metals such as copper and lead, bad odor, "hardness" and nitrates.
- Ion exchange, a system in which the positive and negative charges of various resins attract iron, nitrates, "hardness" and trace metals out of the water.
- Distillation, a process that removes "hardness," trace metals, odor, hydrogen sulfide (the "rotten egg" smell in some water), nitrates, bacteria and iron by heating water until it turns to

steam, then condensing it back into water again.

- Chlorination.
- Manganese green-sand filtration, a system that works much like an ion exchanger except that it uses only green-sand—a naturally occurring material—as a filter.

Periodically, of course, all of these systems need to be cleaned or flushed to remain effective.

Be sure to follow the manufacturer's instructions on the system you buy. Or if you don't want the hassle of maintaining a water-treatment system, buy bottled water instead for drinking and cooking. One out of every 17 Americans already does.

MAKE IT CLEAN

But keeping our homes healthy involves more than just getting rid of indoor air and water pollution. It also means getting rid of the germs and molds that can make us sick, particularly if we have allergies or asthma. How can we protect ourselves from these common molds, pollens, mites, fungi and algae that are known to affect our health?

Fortunately, the job isn't too complicated, says Michael Lebowitz, Ph.D., professor of internal medicine at the University of Arizona Medical Center.

One way, he says, is with an air filtration device. Another is ensuring proper humidity—too damp or too dry and those creepy creatures and growths can have a field day. If your house is too damp, a dehumidifier will help. If it's too dry, you can use a humidifier. In either case, clean the machines. And we're not talking every spring. The American Lung Association suggests a once-over with mild soap and water every 24 hours.

MAKE YOUR JOB A BIT HEALTHIER

But a safe, healthy environment should not start and stop at your front door. At work, ice machines,

water coolers, air conditioning duct-work and cooling towers should be scrubbed out periodically. And you should feel perfectly comfortable asking your custodial staff or building engineer to do it. After all, they're as likely to get sick from moldy oldies in the ducts as you are.

Indoor pollution doesn't stop on your doorstep, either. Studies indicate that radon isn't as much of a problem in large public buildings as it is in the small, confined spaces of our homes, but asbestos—which is usually found only as a sealant for fireplaces and heating ducts in our homes—can be a significant problem at work.

Asbestos is a fireproof insulating material that produces airborne fibers that, when inhaled, can cause cancer and fibrous tissue growth in the lungs.

An EPA report states that "no level of exposure is considered without significant risk." So if you suspect there is asbestos in your workplace—or if you find white fibrous dust on your desk or work station—report it to the nearest branch of the National Institute for Occupational Safety and Health (NIOSH), the Occupational Safety and Health Administration or the U.S. Department of Labor.

Under no circumstances should you disturb the suspected material, experts suggest. (See "Asbestos Handling Is for Professionals")

IS YOUR WORKPLACE SICK?

Air pollution in the workplace is not limited to asbestos. But it's usually solved more easily. Studies on office pollution have found methyl alcohol in the air from spirit duplicators such as mimeograph machines, butyl methacrylate from facsimile recorders that send photocopies over telephone lines, ammonia from blueprint machines, formaldehyde from carbonless copy paper and urea formaldehyde from wall insulation.

Sounds terrible, doesn't it? And workers were miserable. Complaints of noxious odors, headaches, eye irritation, dizziness and lethargy were common. But the solution,

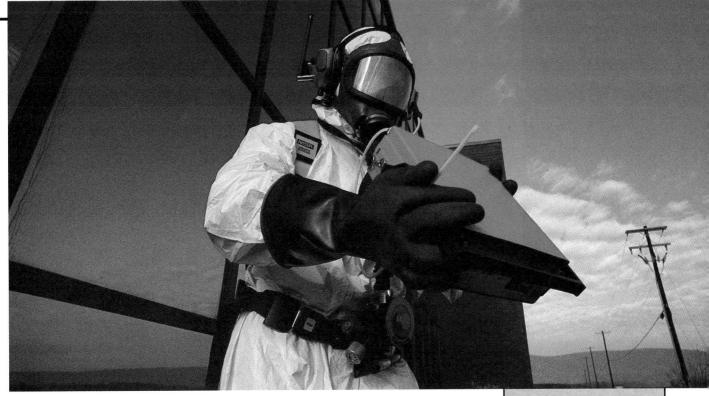

investigators concluded, was devastatingly simple: They provided several of the office machines with local exhausts, moved workers away from others, increased ventilation and turned on the ventilating systems before workers arrived in the morning.

Simple, right? Essentially all they did was move the air around. And the problems and their easy resolution are typical. A study of 203 indoor air-quality complaints investigated by NIOSH, for example, reveals that nearly a third of the reported headache-fatigue-nausea-dizziness problems were caused by formaldehyde and other chemicals. But according to Jim Melius, M.D., chief of hazard evaluation and technical assistance for NIOSH in Cincinnati, the problem—which has since come to be known as sick-building syndrome—was triggered by inadequate ventilation in almost *half* of NIOSH's investigations.

As British researchers concluded in a separate study, sick-building syndrome may very well be caused by a workplace practice that keeps energy costs down by recirculating up to 90 percent of a building's air.

Clearly, the solution is to avoid such a temptation, says Dr. Melius. And if smokers are allowed to light up in the workplace, the amount of outside air drawn into the office or factory should be quadrupled, say other experts.

But the National Academy of Sciences goes one step further, suggesting that employers consider restricting or banning smoking in the workplace.

SMOKERS UNITE!

No smoking in buildings and offices? Is it really necessary to kick out the smokers?

The academy is probably responding to studies that demonstrate the effects of tobacco smoke on nonsmokers. One such study of 2,100 adults, for example, revealed lung impairment in nonsmokers who worked for 20 years or more in offices where smoking was permitted. Tragically, the nonsmokers lost as much lung capacity as if they had smoked 10 cigarettes a day themselves for at least 20 years.

It's one thing if you decide to smoke yourself; it's another to force others to inhale as well.

That's the focal point of an argument that has ended up in courts, state legislatures and town councils more than once. The state of

Asbestos Handling Is for Professionals

There is *no* safe level of exposure to asbestos, says the EPA. It should be removed—a job for professionals wearing full protective gear, including respirators.

Asbestos also can be temporarily enclosed on all sides or encapsulated within a special sprayed-on substance, provided the material is in good shape and not near a building's occupants.

Washington, for example, requires no-smoking areas in all workplaces. In New Jersey, workplaces that accommodate 50 or more employees are required to establish in-house rules that protect the health, welfare and comfort of employees from the detrimental effects of tobacco smoke.

The message is not just, "Don't smoke around *us,* you turkey!" It's also, "We love you—enough to want you to quit."

Individual smokers who quit are often given a lot of support from their co-workers. When Janet decided to quit, for example, her fellow workers not only encouraged her, they also donated "prizes" for succeeding: one month of free lunches in the corporate dining room, a case of her favorite beverage, a professional manicure, a lucky stone won in a sweepstakes lottery, a food store gift certificate and a hand-crocheted Christmas stocking.

Clearly, a smoke-free workplace doesn't *have* to be a confrontative, hostile, smoker-vs.-nonsmoker environment. It can also be a caring, healthful place.

MAKE IT QUIET

But even if your air is as clean as you can possibly make it, there's one more airborne problem to solve before your work environment can shelter, stimulate and nourish. And that problem is noise.

Noise is actually any sound that annoys or displeases you. At its worst—when you risk hearing loss—it's a jet engine or a jackhammer or a live rock band. At its best, it's the rustle of a leaf. But there's a whole range of sound in between that can still drive you wild. And when it does, the results, scientists say, can be impaired thinking, increased aggression and a reduced tolerance of the differences between you and other people.

So how do you keep it quiet?

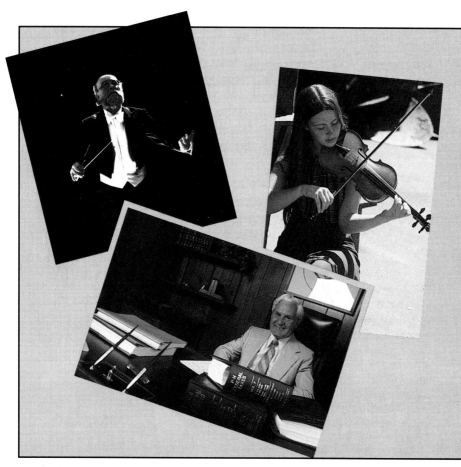

Healthy Jobs, Unhealthy Jobs

The most healthful occupations may be those that require a physical workout, says Hans H. Neumann, M.D., a former medical director of the health department in New Haven, Connecticut. Orchestra conductors, violinists and pianists, for example, all perform physically demanding activities that, researchers say, may condition the cardiovascular system as the performers work.

Ironically, some of the most unhealthful occupations all generally involve intense physical activity, too—but of a risky nature. Logging, ship-

Numerous devices ranging from solid rubber ear plugs to acoustical ear muffs are available. You can also block out noisy co-workers with headphones plugged into a cassette player. A Gregorian chant, a Sousa march or a Puccini opera can go a long way toward shutting out even the loudest and least considerate of people.

BLOCK IT, STIFLE IT, STOP IT

You can also block noise by moving furniture such as bookcases against the walls of noisy rooms to absorb sound, laying rugs and padding over hardwood or tile floors, setting up space dividers and asking for acoustical ceilings when the company remodels. Heavy draperies are also good noise-stoppers, as are acoustical pads under typewriters, masking tape on telephone bells and plastic covers or shields over computer printers.

But workplace health means more than stifling noisy co-workers and typewriters, isolating smokers while encouraging them to quit, venting machinery or airing out buildings.

If you sit, it also means a good chair with back support, an adjustable armrest and a wide padded seat made of porous, textured material.

If you stand, it means keeping your weight evenly distributed on both feet.

It means special glasses, glare shields, hourly rest breaks, flexible screens and detachable keyboards if you use a VDT.

And for every worker in every job, it means plastic shields on fluorescent lights and the use of task lighting—lighting that's really appropriate for the work being done—whenever possible.

But above all, home and workplace health means valuing yourself enough to pay attention to the world that surrounds you. It means mastering your personal environment. And you can.

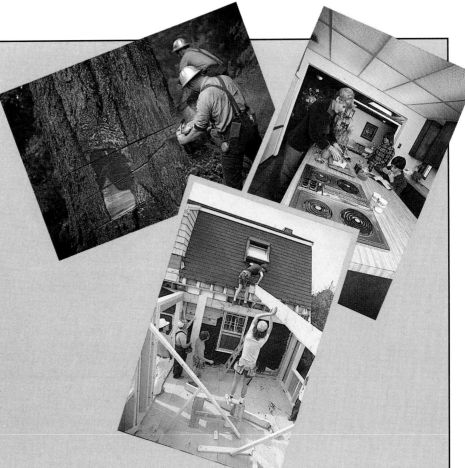

building and roofing are not three occupations you would choose for those near and dear. One surprise among unhealthful occupations, however, is homemaking. And we're not talking dishpan hands. Studies of cancer and work show homemakers have the highest job-related cancer death rate. Unfortunately, nobody quite knows why.

Experts do know why executives enjoy some of the best heart health in America—the theory is that because they're in control of their work flow and job assignments, their stress levels are low.

6

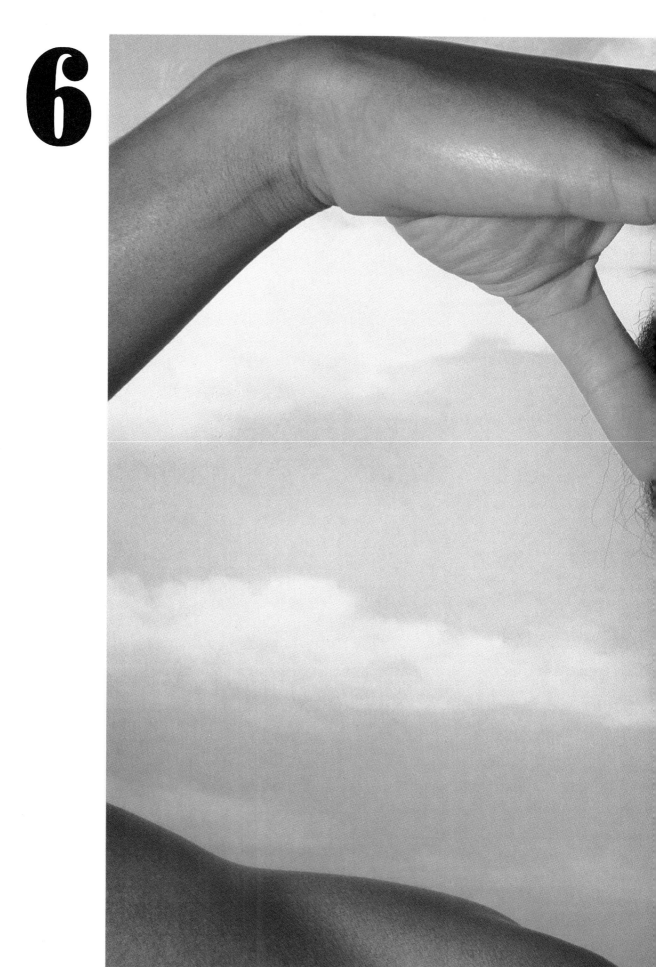

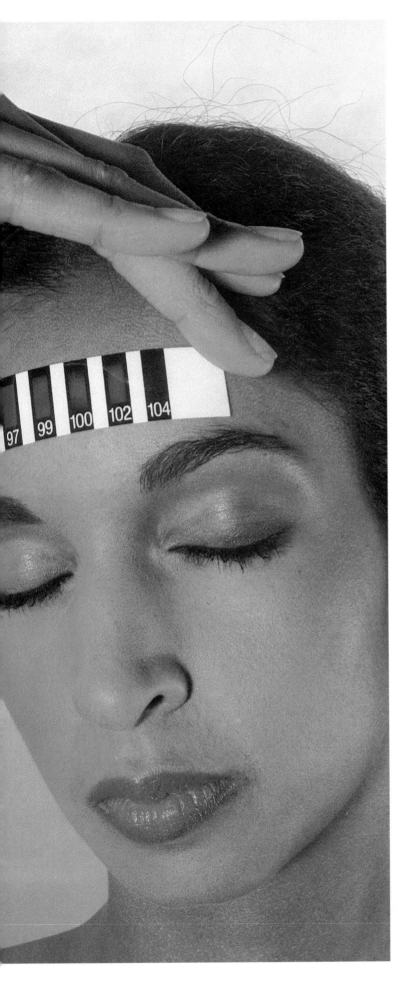

Mastering Self-Care

Do-it-yourself medicine has come of age as people literally "take care of number one!"

Flashback to 1970. A year has passed since a man walked on the moon. Pocket calculators are the rage. The reign of the computer chip is well under way. Technology is advancing at warp speed. It's the dawn of a bold new era.

Or is it?

Self-care pioneer Keith W. Sehnert, M.D., is having trouble getting medical equipment for students in his patient-education series. He advises his Washington, D.C., patients to buy their own stethoscopes and blood pressure cuffs to monitor their blood pressures. But none of the area medical supply stores will sell the cherished "tools of the gods" to the unwashed. Dr. Sehnert cleverly resorts to giving his patients his own stethoscope and advising them to wear it into the store. Effectively disguised as doctors or nurses, they are sold the equipment without any questions asked.

At Yale Medical School, Lowell Levin, Ed.D., M.P.H., has just returned from an eye-opening trip to Great Britain. He found British doctors swamped with patients complaining about trivial problems. He views it as a warning for America. The way to avoid this situation is obvious—self-care.

Although determined to spread the word, he meets resistance from an often-hostile medical community. "I can't even get a paper published," he laments. Disappointed, he considers giving up.

But he doesn't. And neither do Dr. Sehnert and a handful of other self-care pioneers. Although they don't know it, they are the flickers of fire dancing off a fuse.

BOOM! The fuse sparks an explosion in the 1980s. Suddenly the idea of self-care becomes a national obsession.

Stores are now begging Joe Average to buy those same blood pressure kits that Dr. Sehnert's patients had to use deceit to acquire. And Joe's buying—more than $200 million worth a year. The entire self-care industry has rocketed from practically nothing to a business that is expected to bring in an estimated $10 billion a year by 1990. With corporate giants such as Sears and Norelco

Digital Diagnostics

Imagine the police lab boys dusting for prints at a murder scene. They conclude: "It's 'Jake the Snake' all right, but better get him quick. His prints say he may soon suffer from Alzheimer's disease."

Don't laugh. Researchers say it may be possible to detect people at high risk for Alzheimer's disease and breast cancer by the whorls and loops in their fingerprints. The patterns are too complicated for self-tests, but you may want to ask your doctor to play Dick Tracy at your next visit.

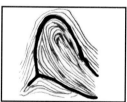
Radial Loop

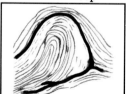
Ulnar Loop

jumping onto the money wagon, that lofty figure may well double.

The boom continues. Almost 200 home medical test kits are now available, with more being devised each day. Fifty self-care newsletters and magazines have sprung up. Dr. Levin stopped counting when the book list grew to 5,000.

Some medical and nursing schools, including those at Yale and the University of Southern California, are now placing a great emphasis on self-care. Offerings are diverse and include services and products such as home intravenous antibiotic therapy, weather prediction services geared to physical and behavioral effects, giant self-help conventions and—for the blind—voice-synthesized blood glucose tests.

So what happened between 1970 and 1980? And just what is self-care?

I, THE DOCTOR

"Good questions," muses Dr. Levin. "Self-care, as I see it, refers to those things individuals and families do for themselves in the areas of promoting health, preventing disease, treating minor illness and injury, managing chronic disease, and rehabilitation."

Dr. Sehnert, author of two books on self-care, adds that some form of layman education is required.

"Self-care is learning to handle everyday health problems with *formal* training in place of the traditional informal training. This means classes, books, course guides or other easy-to-understand sources."

Out West, where self-care is really surging, Tom F. Griffin, Jr., M.D., of Douglas, Arizona, agrees with Dr. Sehnert's educational approach.

"A lot of resistance to self-care is based on fear and intimidation. People don't have a basic understanding of how the body works. Most people know how their cars and toilets work better than their own bodies. Once you have a basic understanding of your body, you should be able to treat your own minor illnesses and problems due to stress and environment."

Is this a bold new concept?

Hardly. Studies in America and Britain found that 65 to 85 percent of all medical care is and has been self-care. Now it has been refined, supported, commercialized and allowed out of the closet.

Dr. Levin also credits the women's health movement, which was responding to growing unrest among women about being abused in a male-dominated medical society. Women began providing for themselves the care they felt they weren't getting from their doctors.

"When they took the speculum out of the hands of the gynecologist and put it into the hands of the women themselves, it was more than the transfer of technology; it was a dramatic challenge to the established health-care system. It also ignited the self-care movement," Dr. Levin feels.

Dr. Sehnert adds two other factors—a growing desire among older people to live healthier lives, and the army of baby boomers who brought their antiestablishment views from the 1960s and applied them to the medical establishment of the 1980s.

Whatever the cause, the boom has delighted the pioneers who struggled so hard in the beginning.

"I think it's wonderful," says Edward R. Pinckney, M.D., coauthor of the book *Do-It-Yourself Medical Testing.* "People are going to prevent an awful lot of illnesses. When people discover they can do something about their health, they take better care of themselves."

"I'm never satisfied, but I am amazed," Dr. Levin adds. "It has been an astounding pattern of growth. I'm surprised by the small amount of negative resistance from the health professionals today. They were the ones who hadn't shared the information in the first place. But by and large, their reaction has been positive."

Dr. Sehnert sees the growth continuing over the next few decades.

"I see it expanding in concentric circles like the ripples of a rock in a pond. There will not be as much dominance of traditional scientific medicine in the future as we have had in the past," he believes. "People, as their own self-care practitioners, will sample other types of healing, such as chiropractic, acupuncture, acupressure, homeopathy, herbal medicines, naturopathy (natural healing avoiding drugs and surgery) and some even more esoteric methods such as energy medicine and spiritual healing."

DOES SELF-CARE WORK?

Enough talk. Is the self-care boom really keeping people healthier? Let's look at some cold, hard numbers.

A survey of 1,004 breast cancer patients performed by Roger S. Foster, Jr., M.D., director of the Vermont Regional Cancer Center, revealed that 90 percent of the afflicted women who had performed breast self-exams detected their own tumors. Moreover, doctors estimated treatment was started a crucial six months earlier for those women than for women who did not regularly examine their breasts. Those who found the tumors had a five-year survival rate of 75 percent, compared to 57 percent for nonexaminers.

At the Ulster Cancer Foundation in Belfast, Northern Ireland, a study of 27,805 women similarly showed that breast self-examination can be an effective self-care tool. In this study, one group of women received from their doctors a booklet encouraging breast exams. A second group—a control group—did not. At the end of the study the doctors concluded that the booklet "is likely to lead to detection of breast cancer at an earlier stage." A second finding was that the booklet had a "modest positive effect" on how quickly women reported to their doctors when they found a lump.

A study by Donald M. Vickery, M.D., director of the Center for Corporate Health Promotion in Reston, Virginia, showed that people who are offered information on total body self-care, such as books, pamphlets, a telephone information service or counseling, made 35 percent fewer medical visits for minor illnesses than members of a control group.

A similar study conducted by doctors at the Family Medical Care Center of the University of Missouri found that people who learned which

A Big Byte of Health

The stereotypical computer freak is usually portrayed as mushy, gray skinned, and all brain, no muscle. Not quite a picture of health. That's odd, because the computer market is teeming with self-care programs on health, fitness and nutrition, as well as other medical information. In addition, software companies are producing new health and fitness programs, covering everything from diets to jogging tips and complete exercise programs. To keep up, check the reviews in the computer magazines (*Popular Computing, Family Computing,* and so on).

cold symptoms signal the need for a doctor's visit and which do not made 44 percent fewer "unnecessary" visits to doctors than members of a control group.

Fewer doctor visits mean more money stays in your pocket! And a study at Kaiser Permanente Hospital in San Diego showed just that. Testing the effects of home blood glucose monitoring for diabetics, researchers concluded that yearly physician visits dropped 79 percent, emergency room visits fell 54 percent and hospital stays plunged 87 percent.

How accurate are the home self-test kits, one of the fastest-growing areas of self-care? "As a whole, I'd say they were 90 percent accurate," says Dr. Pinckney. "Some, like the blood pressure kits and home pregnancy tests, when properly used, are close to 99 percent accurate. On the lower end, the urea nitrogen [kidney disease] blood tests are about 80 percent accurate, as are the breath alcohol tests the police give. The test for occult blood in the feces is only about 70 percent accurate, and if you take large doses of vitamin C, it can

(continued on page 72)

Self-Care Kits

It started quietly with EPTs—Early Pregnancy Test kits sold directly to the consumer. Then, before you could say "megabucks," the market became swamped with self-care kits.

"The tests are quite accurate," says Edward Pinckney, M.D., a proponent of home self-testing. "The market for these tests is going to continue to grow. People will soon go to their doctor not to ask, 'what's wrong?' but to say, 'This is what I've found, now what can we do about it?' The illnesses and diseases can be detected much earlier and may enable doctors to cure them faster. Just remember to follow the directions precisely and, if possible, do each test at least twice, rereading the directions each time." That's to make sure you don't become emotionally upset about a false reaction, or make a procedural mistake that either causes a false reaction or prevents a positive reaction."

Venereal Disease

This is a partial home test kit for gonorrhea, for men only. A discharge sample is placed on a glass slide and allowed to dry, then placed in the mailing case provided and mailed to the company laboratory. Results may be learned by calling the laboratory.

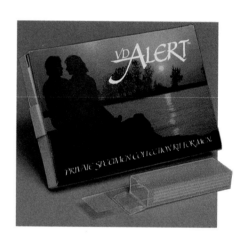

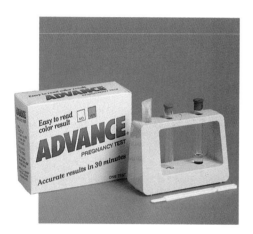

Pregnancy

This was the first type of home self-test kit. It tells a woman whether or not she is pregnant by detecting the pregnancy hormone human chorionic gonadotropin in urine. It includes a dipstick, a plastic vial containing buffer solution, glass tubes, dried test chemicals, color-developing solution, a test stand, a color chart and a urine collection container.

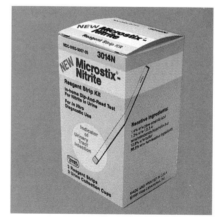

Urinary Tract Infections

This is an extremely simple test to reveal the presence of bacterial infections. Materials include dipsticks, a urine collection cup and a color chart.

Condition	Test Kit Brand Name	
Blood glucose	Visidex II	
Colorectal disorders	Early Detector	
Ovulation	OvuSTICK	
Pregnancy	Advance	
Urinary glucose	Clinistix	
Urinary tract infections	Microstix-Nitrite	
Venereal disease	VD Alert	

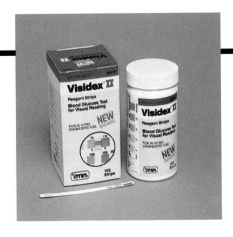

Blood Glucose

This test checks glucose levels in the blood, basically for diabetics. After pricking a finger (the manufacturer advises buying a special sterilized device for this purpose), the tester places a drop of blood on a pair of tiny reaction pads set on a strip of plastic, blots the sample, then compares it with a color chart. There are two tests involved.

Colorectal Disorders

This test detects blood in the stool, which can be an early sign of many colorectal disorders, including hemorrhoids, ulcerative colitis, diverticulosis, polyps and cancer. After a stool smear is obtained on a pad, a special developer solution is sprayed on the smear. A resulting blue color is an indication of blood in the stool.

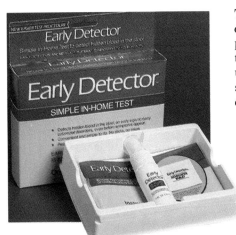

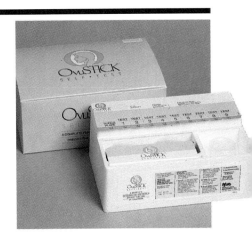

Ovulation

This test pinpoints the time of ovulation to enhance the chance of pregnancy. It works by detecting the luteinizing hormone in the urine. Materials include test tubes, stoppers, vials, powders, solutions, dipsticks and a color chart.

Results Time	Cost (subject to change)	Manufacturer
30 seconds 90 seconds	100 strips for $55	Ames Division Miles Laboratories, Inc., P.O. Box 70, Elkhart, IN 46515
30-60 seconds	$7	Warner-Lambert Co. Morris Plains, NJ 07950
1 hour	$60	Monoclonal Antibodies, Inc. 2319 Charleston Road, Mountain View, CA 94043
30 minutes	$10-$12 (per procedure)	Advanced Care Products Ortho Pharmaceutical Corp. Raritan, NJ 08869
10 seconds	50 dipsticks for $4.35	Ames Division Miles Laboratories, Inc. P.O. Box 70, Elkhart, IN 46515
Immediately	3 strips and materials for $3.49	Ames Division Miles Laboratories, Inc. P.O. Box 70, Elkhart, IN 46515
Approximately 48 hours after slide arrives at the lab	$15-$19	Medical Frontiers, Inc. Centerville, OH 45459

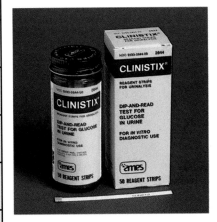

Urinary Glucose

This is a simple, dip-and-read test to chart the levels of glucose (sugar) in the urine and measure carbohydrate metabolism. Basically for diabetics, it uses dipsticks and a color chart.

71

give you a false negative, meaning you could be bleeding and it will not detect it."

Overall, Dr. Pinckney's 90 percent rate would seem to exceed the accuracy rate of tests performed by labs or doctors, which is 86 percent.

Are the basic concepts of self-care difficult to practice?

Charles E. Lewis, M.D., professor of internal medicine at the University of California School of Medicine, Los Angeles, decided to find out. He set up a three-year program among elementary school students, some as young as five years old, that gave them control of their own health care by allowing them to decide when they needed to visit the school nurse and even choose their own treatment when they got there. Dr. Lewis concluded that the children were "enormously competent at self-care" and were especially adept at pinpointing stress as the cause of numerous ailments.

TREATING YOURSELF

Before you start patting yourself on your strong, healthy, self-treated back, here's another view on the subject.

"The self-care boom is a fraud," declares Gershon Lesser, M.D., clinical professor of medicine at the University of Southern California.

"I hear more people talk a good game of self-care than talk about the big fish that got away. Talk is cheap. If self-care was booming, the tobacco industry and alcohol industry would be bankrupt. The biggest medical breakthrough of modern times has yet to occur. That is the massive awareness that the primary responsibility for health lies with the patient."

"I might not go as far as saying it's a 'fraud,'" counters Roger Seehafer, Ph.D., a professor of health education at Purdue University. However, being in California, where the fads are incredibly superficial, Dr. Lesser

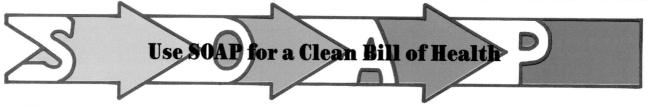

Use SOAP for a Clean Bill of Health

Here's an easy way to practice self-treatment. The key word to remember is SOAP.

Devised by Lawrence L. Weed, M.D., of South Burlington, Vermont, the SOAP system is currently being taught in corporate seminars by self-care pioneer Keith W. Sehnert, M.D.

"The *S* stands for *subjective*," Dr. Sehnert explains. "It means learning to describe your illness or injury, the who, what, when and where of your symptoms." Instead of "I have a headache," learn to say, "I have a frontal headache that hurts only when I bend over."

The *O* stands for *objective*, and calls for an objective measurement of your symptoms. "Diarrhea ten times a day is one thing; diarrhea four times a day is another," says Dr. Sehnert. Knowing how

to take vital signs—pulse, respiration, temperature, blood pressure—is extremely helpful.

A is for *assessment*. You size up the problem and decide what to do. Two good books that take you step by step through nearly every illness are Dr. Sehnert's *How to Be Your Own Doctor (Sometimes)*, and *Take Care of Yourself: A Consumer's Guide to Medical Care*, by Donald M. Vickery, M.D., and James F. Fries, M.D.

The final *P* is for *plan*. Set up a treatment plan for yourself and stick to it! "Say to yourself, I'll try this home treatment for 2 days. If I'm not better by then, I'll go to a doctor," Dr. Sehnert advises. If you are relying on over-the-counter medications, pay close attention to the time limitations on the label.

may be right on the money for his area. "What I see overall is that the public has indeed become acutely aware of exactly what steps need to be taken to live healthier, disease-free lives. They are just unwilling or not yet ready to assume the responsibility and discipline required to change their lifestyles. This will take longer," Dr. Seehafer says.

What both Dr. Seehafer and Dr. Lesser are saying is that you can't practice preventive health and self-treatment vicariously. Buying a health book, paging through it, then stashing it away is shelf-care, not self-care. Self-care requires self-action.

The first self-action is to know what you can safely treat and what remains the province of your doctor.

A survey taken by a professional opinion-research company determined that 85 percent of the American population currently uses self-care to treat problems identified as minor pain or injury, indigestion, coughs and colds, sore throats, skin infections, acne, allergies and arthritis pain.

However, before you go to the medicine cabinet to treat these and other minor illnesses, be aware of signals that warn you that the problem is out of your league.

"You should consult a physician if you cough up or vomit blood, or notice a black or bloody stool," advises Tom Ferguson, M.D., another self-care pioneer. "See a doctor if you notice yellowing in the whites of your eyes; a sore that doesn't heal; a breast lump; or an unexplained thickening anywhere in your body. Also if you experience a marked and unexplained weight loss, sudden shortness of breath or any dramatic change in your normal body functioning. Go to a doctor immediately if you suffer a crushing pain in the chest that may be accompanied by pain radiating down the left arm, nausea, clammy skin, difficulty in breathing or an irregular heartbeat. Call the doctor immediately if you or your child receives a blow on the head that causes unconsciousness or has abdominal pain that lasts for 2 hours or more or is very intense for several hours," he says.

Free of those symptoms, here are two typical problems that Dr. Sehnert says you can treat, along with how to treat them.

The Common Cold. "Colds last from three to seven days, with a gradual one- or two-day onset. Low-grade fever usually occurs on the third day, with full-blown symptoms for about three days. After the third day, symptoms should gradually subside," Dr. Sehnert explains.

What to do. "Avoid excessively cold temperatures and overfatigue. Go to bed if you have a fever. Get extra rest. Increase your liquid intake to about 8 ounces of juice or water every 2 hours. Stop smoking. Gargle with hot salt water. Use throat lozenges and nose drops if they help. Use a nasal decongestant—pill or tablet, not spray—if needed. Take aspirin if needed. Check your temperature three times daily and record it."

When to call the doctor. "You should see a doctor if you have a temperature over 101 degrees several times each day; increasing throat pain, white or yellow spots on the tonsils or throat; shaking chills and chattering teeth; chest pain; shortness of breath; earache; pain in the sinuses; coughing that produces colored sputum; or no improvement by the fifth day," Dr. Sehnert says.

Cuts and Wounds. "Lacerations can easily be treated at home, but many people, not knowing the guidelines, become frightened and make unnecessary trips to health-care practitioners." Dr. Sehnert explains.

What to do. "Apply direct pressure with any clean cloth available to control the bleeding. Keep the pressure on for 3 minutes before you look. If bleeding isn't a problem, apply ice (in a plastic bag) or cold water for about 10 minutes to minimize swelling. If the wound is dirty, wash it with clean water and mild soap. Make sure that particles of dirt, sand, glass, etc., have been flushed out by running water on [the wound] for about 5 minutes. Apply an antibacterial ointment and dress the wound. Change the dressing in 24 hours. The wound should be kept dry, dressed, protected and immobilized for one week," Dr. Sehnert recommends.

When to call the doctor. "Call a doctor if there is a gaping wound more than 1 inch long; persistent bleeding and blood soaking through the dressing; temperature over 100 degrees; numbness below the wound; red streaks radiating away from the wound; persistent and increasing pain; inability to move a joint below the wound; swollen nodes in the leg, groin, armpit or neck; if the laceration is caused by a human or animal bite; if the wound is a puncture and lockjaw (tetanus) is a possibility (as in a 'dirty' outdoor wound, farm accidents, rust, etc.)."

For a complete, detailed description of how to treat the most common illnesses, injuries and emergencies, consult either or both of Dr. Sehnert's books, *How to Be Your Own Doctor (Sometimes),* revised edition, and *Selfcare/Wellcare.*

STAYING ALIVE

The most important aspect of self-care is not treating the small illnesses, it's preventing the big killer diseases. And this is an area where your role is vital.

First, some more warnings.

"People assume they can abuse themselves with impunity because they'll be rescued by the new medical techniques and technology. I've got news for those people. No medical breakthroughs have justified a life of installment-plan self-destruction." says Dr. Lesser, who is also an attorney. "Smoking, drinking, abusive sex, drugs, junk foods, fatty foods, obesity, sedentary lifestyles completely lacking exercise—they all mean cancer, heart disease, deadly social diseases like AIDS, and a host of other killers. And don't come to us doctors. We haven't got the cures. Your life is in your hands."

Dr. Lesser has a unique way of turning people on to self-care. He uses a "scared straight" technique similar to that used by juvenile authorities who bus children and teenagers to prisons to experience firsthand what life behind bars is really like. Dr. Lesser brings the kids to the cancer wards of local hospitals.

"You show them the people in agony, wasting away in pain, dying from their abuses. Then you tell them, 'Take a good look. One in three

people now gets cancer. If you want to end up here, okay. If you don't, then here are the things you can do.' "

The beauty of the self-care plan to prevent major disease is that it's easy. No thick medical books or expensive tools are needed. Unless you have the will power of a mashed potato, you should be able to avoid the bad habits Dr. Lesser mentioned, or kick them if you currently are hooked.

Need more convincing? A few years ago the United States Surgeon General said, "Seven of the ten leading causes of death in the United States could be substantially reduced through commonsense changes in the lifestyles of many Americans." The areas of change were identified in the report as diet, smoking, exercise, alcohol abuse and use of hypertension medication. The use of seat belts and other auto safety precautions has now been added to the list.

Dr. Seehafer sums up the simple, antidisease self-care plan this way. "If you smoke, quit. If you drink, do so in moderation. If you are obese, diet. And everyone should exercise regularly." To prevent serious accidents, he says, "If you're taking a drive, buckle up. If you're using a motorcycle, wear a helmet."

PROBLEMS OF SELF-TESTING

Studies around the world have shown that one of the most promoted methods of self-care—breast self-examination for women—has proven beyond doubt to be a lifesaver. But despite these positive results and the fact that 1 in 11 women develops breast cancer, a recent Gallup survey on behalf of the American Institute for Cancer Research determined that nearly *two-thirds* of the women polled are still not performing the recommended monthly examinations. And this was despite the fact that 95 percent said they had heard of breast self-exam.

Even among women performing the exams, another study found a shockingly large percentage are doing them wrong. Sheryle Alagna, Ph.D., of the medical psychology department of the Uniformed Services University of the Health Sciences in Bethesda, Maryland, tested 73 women by asking them to locate tumors on a life-size torso that duplicated human breasts. Seven tumors were planted in the artificial breasts—four superficial and three deeply embedded. Incredibly, only 1 woman found all seven, and 5 women didn't find any!

This test is so important, all women should know how to do it right. Here's how:

Observe your breasts in the mirror for skin pulling, dimpling, nipples scaling or crusting or any watery, yellow, pink or bloody discharge.

Lean forward slightly to observe any changes in the breasts, like skin puckering.

Raise your arms slowly overhead. Examine the breasts for changes.

Then rest your raised hands against your forehead. Observe any changes.

Next, tighten your chest and arm muscles. Again, look for changes.

Lie down on your back with a folded towel under your right shoulder and your right arm tucked around your head. With your left hand cupped, use the flat of your fingers to feel for lumps or skin changes in your right breast. In a rotary direction, examine the inner half of the right breast from the collarbone to the underportion and from the nipple to the breastbone. Then examine the outer area between the nipple and the armpit (including the armpit itself), where most cancers occur. (A ridge of firm tissue in the lower curve of each breast is normal.) Repeat the steps, using the right hand to feel the left breast.

Men, you have an important self-test, too. Testicular cancer is not common, yet it is *the* most common solid tumor found in men between the ages of 20 and 34, according to Marc B. Garnick, M.D., and Robert J. Mayer, M.D., of the Sidney Farber Cancer Institute, Boston. They recommend that men perform a testicular self-examination with the same diligence and frequency as women do breast exams.

The best time to perform the simple 3-minute self-exam is right

Tom Ferguson, M.D.: Self-Care Pioneer

"Dr. Ferguson, after being a doctor all these years, have you applied for your license to practice medicine yet?"

"No. And I don't think it's likely."

That sums up Tom Ferguson's attitude. While he is a fullfledged M.D., he never took the final, and probably easiest, step in his grueling medical training. The reason is that, instead of practicing medicine, Dr. Ferguson has a greater calling—teaching people to take care of *themselves*. His "practice" is limited to speeches, lectures, putting out his own publication, *Medical Self-Care* magazine, and writing self-care books.

"My fellow medical students at Yale thought I was crazy," Dr. Ferguson recalls. "The idea of self-care was rather obscure in 1975. Now it is heard all the time and receives wide support."

Much of this acceptance and support is due to Dr. Ferguson and the innovative magazine, but he feels "two areas need more attention—teaching self-care and self-management skills to children, and the development of tools for psychological self-care. I would hope in the next decade we see similar advances in these fields.

"I don't envision a world without doctors," Dr. Ferguson assures. "I'd like to see a world where doctors are used appropriately."

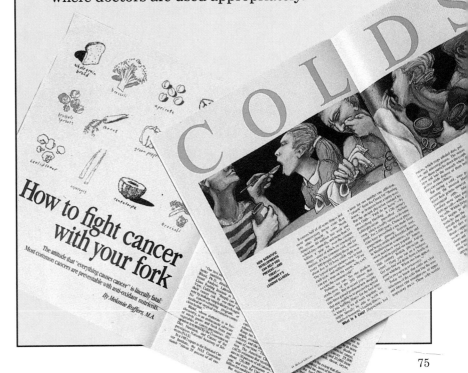

How to fight cancer with your fork

The attitude that "everything causes cancer" is literally fatal! Most common cancers are preventable with anti-oxidant nutrients.

By Melanie Rogers, M.A.

COLDS

The Doctors' Dozen

The experts choose the best self-care books:

Lowell S. Levin, Ed.D., M.P.H., professor of public health, Yale University, recommends:

How to Be Your Own Doctor (Sometimes)
— Keith W. Sehnert, M.D.

The People's Pharmacy, vols. I, II and III
— Joe Graedon

The Medical Show — Editors of Consumer Reports Books

The new *Our Bodies, Ourselves* — Boston's Women's Health Book Collective

Where There Is No Doctor: A Village Health Care Handbook — David Werner

Take Care of Yourself: A Consumer's Guide to Medical Care — Donald M. Vickery, M.D., and James F. Fries, M.D.

Tom Ferguson, M.D., founder of *Medical Self-Care* magazine, recommends:

The Allergy Self-Help Book — Sharon Faelten

Don't Shoot the Dog! — Karen Pryor

Health and Healing: Understanding Conventional and Alternative Medicine — Andrew Weil, M.D.

Messages: The Communication Book — Matthew McKay, Ph.D., Martha Davis, Ph.D., and Patrick Fanning

Menopause, Naturally: Preparing for the Second Half of Life — Sadja Greenwood, M.D., M.P.H.

---

after a warm bath or shower, when the skin of the scrotum is most relaxed. Examine the testicles separately, using the fingers of both hands. Put your index and middle fingers underneath the testicle and your thumb on top. Then gently roll the testicle between the thumb and fingers. (If it hurts, you're applying too much pressure.) A normal testicle is oval and somewhat firm to the touch and should be smooth and free of lumps. On the back side of each testicle you'll feel the epididymis (sperm storage duct), which is a little spongier to the touch.

What you are searching for — and hoping not to find — is a small, hard, usually painless lump or swelling on the front or side of the testicle.

If you find one, have it checked by a doctor immediately.

DO IT YOUR WAY

In addition to these two manual examinations, many self-test kits are available to today's consumer. While most of the tests are reasonably priced, some carry a hefty fee. There is also a host of equally efficient and medically valuable self-tests that have the best price tag of all — free! Most of these freebies require no materials, or rely on things you have around the house.

Dr. Pinckney, who with his wife, Cathey, wrote *Do-It-Yourself Medical Testing,* offers some easy-to-perform tests.

Smell. "As people age they tend to lose their youthful ability to discern odors. This diminished sense is rarely recognized by the deprived individual and could lead to catastrophes if the person fails to detect escaping gas from a stove or heater, smoke from a fire, and even spoiled or contaminated food.

"Here's how to test for smell function. Close your eyes, then have someone open a jar of instant coffee, peel a clove of fresh garlic, break open a chocolate bar and burn a match. (Don't test with ammonia or menthol; they are irritants.) If you fail to detect any of the odors, your doctor can give you a more thorough examination. Loss of smell may be the first indication of a cerebral circulatory problem, concealed cancer, dietary deficiency or depression," explains Dr. Pinckney.

Taste. "Taste function also diminishes with age. Those who have lost the ability to taste have also lost the ability to distinguish spoiled food or dangerous chemicals. Perception of salty flavor can diminish, causing an increased sodium intake. Test for taste by closing your eyes and having someone present you with a bitter flavor (undiluted quinine water), a salty flavor (1 teaspoon of salt dissolved in 4 ounces of water), a sour flavor (1 teaspoon of vinegar dissolved in 1 ounce of water) and a sweet flavor (1 teaspoon of sugar

Building Your Own Self-Care Library

Here's a quick way to build a good home self-care library. Start with the first five books on the "best" list on the opposite page.

To round out the shelves, Maryann Napoli, associate director of the Center for Medical Consumers in New York, suggests these additional publications.

Books: *The Essential Guide to Prescription Drugs; The Essential Guide to Non-Prescription Drugs; How to Raise a Healthy Child. . .In Spite of Your Doctor; Dr. Spock's Baby and Child Care; The Practical Encyclopedia of Natural Healing.*

Magazines: *Nutrition Action* (from the Center for Science and Public Interest, Washington D.C.), *Prevention; Medical Self-Care.*

Newsletters: *Health Facts Newsletter* (from the Center for Medical Consumers in New York).

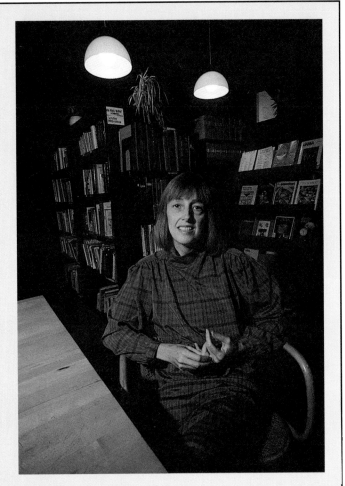

dissolved in 4 ounces of water.) Loss of taste can be an indication of surreptitious drug use or of one of many illnesses or nutritional deficiencies. If you have trouble with the tastes, consult your doctor," Dr. Pinckney says.

Alzheimer's Disease. "Because of media publicity, many people past midlife worry about senile dementia, especially the form known as Alzheimer's disease," says Dr. Pinckney." It can be most comforting for people who are concerned to test themselves, or be tested by some other family member, on a regular basis (every six months or so). One such evaluation can be done with the 'mini-object test.'

"Offer the individual small plastic models of common tools and everyday implements such as a shovel, saw, rake, ladder, rifle, and the like. Ask them to identify the object and explain how it works or what purpose it serves. (You can obtain these objects in a game called Jack Straws, available in toy stores.)

"Award one point for each object recognized and a second point for understanding its use. A perfect score using 15 of the Jack Straws would be 30 points. Anything under 24 points warrants a visit to the doctor. This test can also be performed by the individual themselves," Dr. Pinckney says.

Vision. "A simple vision test involves looking at a lamppost, flagpole or door frame, first with one eye and then with the other," Dr. Pinckney explains. "If the up-and-down line is not straight or complete, or if there is blurring of a segment of the line or pole, medical attention is mandated.

"Remember, these tests, like all home tests, are not for people who already have symptoms or signs of problems. They are for health maintenance. If you have symptoms or signs, it's time to get professional care, not to take a test," Dr. Pinckney warns. "The whole point of most of these tests is to spot the problem before the pain and symptoms come."

Body Gremlins!

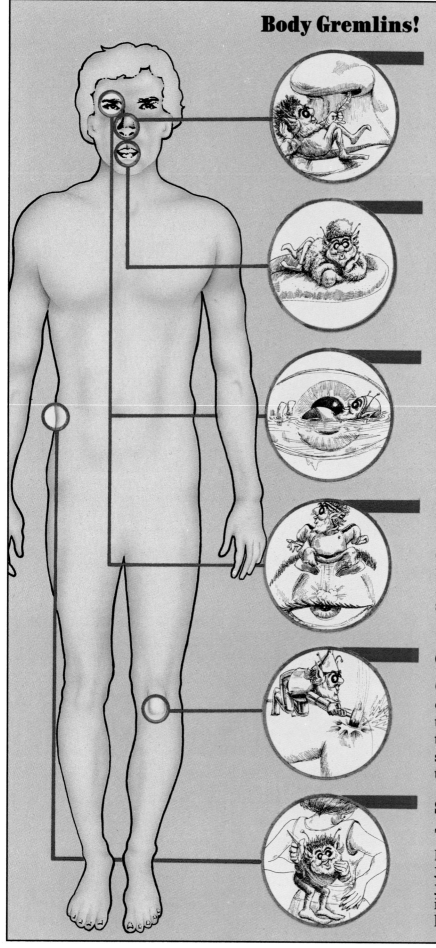

Sudden Sneeze Reflex

Sneezing episodes can occur for any number of reasons—allergies, emotions, sexual excitement, even sunlight. The cure depends on the cause. Find the cause, learn how to handle it, and you're set.

Coated Tongue

An ugly, coated tongue is usually nothing to be alarmed about. The tongue is a notorious cell shedder and the coating is merely dead cells. Color is unimportant.

Floaters

Tiny specks floating across your eye may be disquieting, but they're generally harmless. They are cells or fibers escaping from eye structures. If they become abundant, see an ophthalmologist.

Eye Twitches

Called myokymia, the twitching can be caused by a temporary imbalance in nerves or blood flow. It is often brought on by stress or strain.

Cracking Joints

Clicks and clacks without subsequent pain or grinding sensations are routine. It's all part of the normal process of our bones, sockets and ligaments jostling together.

Side Stitches

The runner's bane, this is the pain that strikes your side when you physically overextend or when you don't warm up before exercising. To ditch the stitch, simply let up and take a rest.

EARLY WARNING SYSTEMS

Here are some more quick, easy tests to uncover an illness in its early stages.

Eyes. Are they bloodshot? This symptom could be a sign of overindulging in alcohol or of swimming too long in chlorinated pools. If your eyes are chronically bloodshot, however, see your doctor. It could be a sign of infection or other disorders.

Here's another test. Gently pull down on one lower eyelid. "The color inside should be pink to dark pink," explains Joseph Ortiz, M.D., an ophthalmologist from Bala Cynwyd, Pennsylvania. "In people who are severely anemic, it's quite white. If that's the case, make sure you get iron in your diet."

Skin. Take a look at your skin. Brown patches (liver spots) or scaly gray patches (keratoses) are signs of sun damage and can develop into cancer. It's best to take care now. Use sunscreens and avoid the mid-day sun.

"Melanoma, a particularly insidious and virulent form of skin cancer, often starts out from slightly raised skin lesions such as a mole or an age spot," warns Herbert Haessler, M.D., of Harvard Medical School. "In the course of enlarging, these spots change from a medium to a dark brown to a bluish or dark gray color. If any skin blemish changes in size, color or texture, it should be evaluated by a doctor without delay."

HELP YOURSELF

Because self-care is the "in" thing in business, medical and governmental circles, the information currently available is staggering. Here are ways to funnel some of this helpful information into your hands.

The U.S. Department of Health and Human Services offers "Health-style," a self-test pamphlet that will enable you to quickly get a handle on your present condition and future needs by answering a series of questions. The pamphlet, and reams of other health information, can be obtained by contacting the National Health Information Clearinghouse, P.O. Box 1133, Washington, DC 20013-1133 (800-336-4797). You can also ask for a resource guide to the self-tests now available.

A wide variety of self-care medical tools and instruments, including "The Home Black Bag" and "The Family Help Kit" can be obtained from the *Medical Self-Care Catalog.* To order a copy, call or write to *Medical Self-Care Catalog,* P.O. Box 999, Pt. Reyes, CA 94956 (415-663-8462).

Self-help groups like Alcoholics Anonymous have expanded geometrically in the 1980s and now number from 50 to 100 even in smaller cities. The groups cover virtually every problem imaginable, including Emotions Anonymous and anorexia and Alzheimer's support groups. For information on the groups in your area, contact the Department of Health and Rehabilitative Services or the local office of the federal Department of Health and Human Services.

To hear taped messages giving information on more than 300 different illnesses and other health issues, ring up Tel-Med. This service is available in about 250 areas of the country. Just call Information in the nearest big city to get the Tel-Med number nearest you.

To receive a newsletter on health issues prepared by the National Action Forum for Mid-Life and Older Women, contact Jane Porcino, Ph.D., Center for Continuing Education, S.B.S., State University of New York, Stony Brook, NY 11794.

Computer junkies can hook into a self-care information system called The Internist. For information write to N-Squared Computing, 5318 Forest Ridge Road, Silverton, OR 97381. Other information clearinghouses include the Self-Help Center, 1600 Dodge Avenue, Evanston, IL 60204 (312-328-0470); the People's Medical Society, 14 East Minor Street, Emmaus, PA 18049 (215-967-2136); and the National Women's Health Network, 224 Seventh Street, SE, Washington, DC 20003 (202-543-9222).

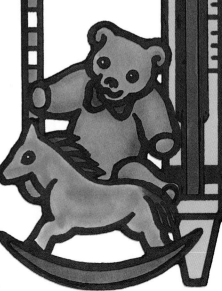

Children's Fevers

- A temperature of 101°F rectally (100°F orally) or above is considered a fever.
- Don't use aspirin or a substitute unless the temperature is 101°F or above.
- Children with flu or chicken pox should not be given aspirin.
- At 103°F or higher, try a lukewarm sponge bath about ½ hour after aspirin or a substitute has been given. Do not use alcohol, because it can be absorbed by the skin and cause seizures.
- 104°F is considered a moderate fever.
- Brain damage does not occur unless the child's fever is higher than 106°F.

7

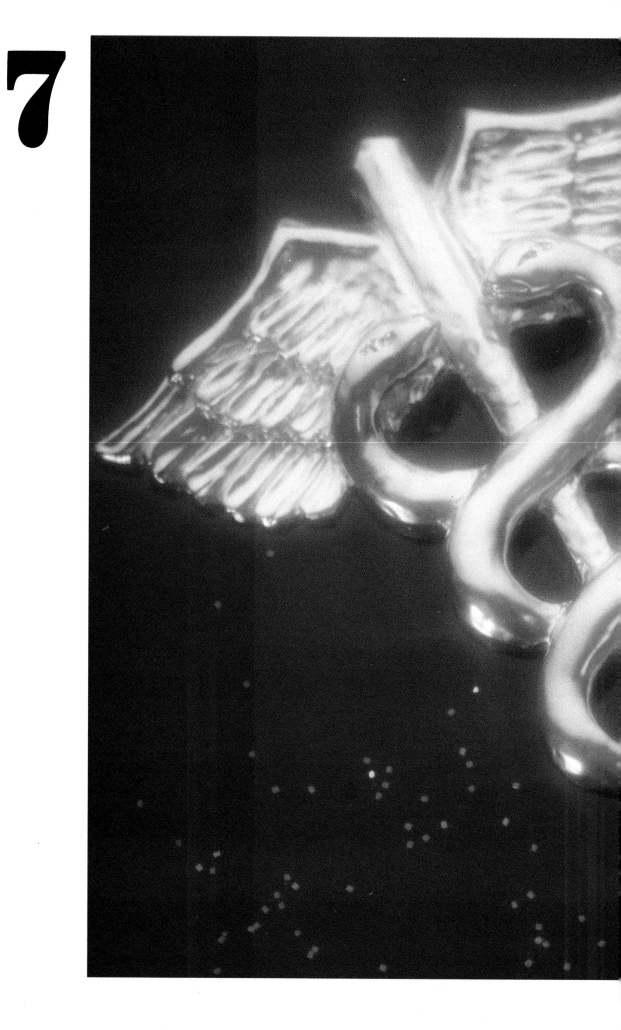

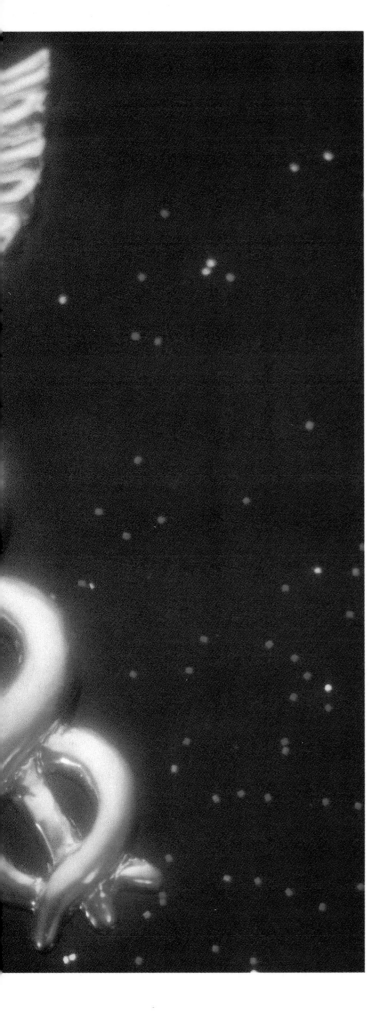

Finding Better Doctors

All doctors are not alike. Here's how to find the good ones and avoid the rest.

Sooner or later, no matter how well you take care of yourself, you're probably going to need help from a member of the medical establishment. Whether the problem is a broken bone, an aching back, an illness or an infection, you want someone both competent and compassionate to help put you back on the road to better health.

Unfortunately, all physicians and health professionals are *not* created equal. Privy to one of the best medical systems in the world, many Americans are nevertheless bitterly disappointed with the medical care they receive.

To avoid disappointment, the wise person learns how to use the system to his advantage. Step one is to choose a good doctor. That choice not only will affect your satisfaction or disappointment with the medical system but also "can mean the difference between life or death for you or some member of your family," points out George D. LeMaitre, M.D., a Massachusetts surgeon and author of *How to Choose a Good Doctor.*

"The Yellow Pages won't tell you which doctors are good and which are bad," says Dr. LeMaitre. "To choose a good doctor, you need to know what to look for."

"You must become a sophisticated consumer," says Lawrence A. May, M.D., in *Getting the Most Out of Your Doctor,* "to avoid being overtested and underinformed."

And you need to know just what *kind* of doctor you're looking for. Is your search for a specialist to treat a specific medical problem? Or do you need a good "primary care" physician to handle everyday medical needs?

The choices are almost endless, but by shopping around and asking the right questions, you can find what you're looking for—a doctor you can trust. With your life.

DOES YOUR DOCTOR PASS THE TEST?

Before you begin your search, it might be a good idea to evaluate the doctor you already have. The "report card" on the opposite page asks the kinds of questions you need to "grade" your personal physician.

Next, compare your doctor's office behavior with the way other physicians treat *their* patients, using the People's Medical Society's (PMS) findings as the basis of comparison. This nonprofit consumer organization asked their members to rate their own doctors, then compiled the results. Their findings give a good indication of what doctors nationwide are doing right—and where improvement is needed.

According to the PMS survey, patients reported that a full 84 percent of their doctors actually *do* take the time to provide a clear, understandable explanation of any tests, treatments or medications that are recommended or prescribed.

However, that figure drops down to only 55 percent when it comes to the number of doctors who include the possibility of potential side effects in that discussion.

Surprisingly, the vast majority of patients felt their bill was within reason, and almost all reported that it was itemized and easily understood.

But 64 percent pointed out that their doctor had failed to discuss which services their insurance would and would not cover—an important issue for those on a limited income.

A majority also noted that they were not informed of the fees prior to their visit, and even more noted that the doctor never discussed the prices of medications, treatments and tests before ordering them.

IS YOUR DOCTOR A TEACHER?

Any failure to discuss fees, side effects or other issues of importance to the patient are warning signs that your doctor may have come down with the most dangerous condition a physician can contract—an inability to communicate with patients.

Like a good teacher, your doctor should explain things clearly—in terms that you'll easily understand—and answer questions directly, not with put-downs or evasions.

Which subjects should be covered? Dr. LeMaitre feels that a good doctor should educate you not only about the best ways to maintain your health and handle your medical problems, including information about any tests or drugs you may need, but also about how your lifestyle directly affects your health and well-being. "A good doctor," he feels, "constantly tries to teach the art of healthy living to his patients."

Why? Because he cares about them as *people,* as well as patients.

"I have never met a doctor who cared for his patients whom I would not trust with my own life," says Dr. LeMaitre. That quality of caring should always be your first criterion in seeking a competent doctor. "After all, you're trying to establish an important human relationship, one that you can safely call upon in moments of severe stress."

Caring can't be measured by some arbitrary index. You have to trust your instincts—pay attention to eye contact and the doctor's responses to your questions.

"The doctor who cares about you is thorough, conscientious, quick to know and admit his own shortcomings and intellectually honest enough to seek the help of specialists if he feels they can contribute to your well-being," says Dr. LeMaitre. He doesn't keep you in the waiting room forever and is available when you need him in an emergency.

He's also a history major. Before a physical exam begins, he should ask detailed questions about your medical history—illnesses, accidents, operations—and that of your family. A complete history will also include a rundown of any drugs you've taken in the past, as well as questions about your work, social habits, alcohol consumption, nutritional status, smoking and the stresses in your life.

A thousand dollars' worth of X rays and blood tests are of little value, says Dr. LeMaitre, without a good history to help the physician understand and interpret them.

(continued on page 88)

Your Doctor's Report Card

1. Did you feel the waiting time at the office was fair and reasonable?
Yes   No   NA

2. Were you treated courteously by the waiting room staff?
Yes   No   NA

3. Did the doctor spend enough time with you?
Yes   No   NA

4. Did the doctor explain any tests, treatments and/or medications that you received?
Yes   No   NA
   a. If no, have you *ever* received such an explanation?
   Yes   No   NA

5. Did the doctor discuss any possible negative side effects of the tests, treatments and/or medications you received?
Yes   No   NA
   a. If no, have you *ever* had such a discussion with your doctor?
   Yes   No   NA

6. Did the doctor discuss his/her qualifications to perform any of the tests or treatments you received?
Yes   No   NA
   a. If no, has this doctor *ever* discussed his/her qualifications to perform a test or treatment?
   Yes   No   NA

7. Did the doctor tell you about any possible pain that might be expected from any of the tests, treatments and/or medications you received?
Yes   No   NA
   a. If no, has this doctor *ever* discussed possible pain that might be expected from any test, treatment and/or medication received?
   Yes   No   NA

Scoring

Add up all the *no* answers. Nobody's perfect, including your doctor—less than 5 *no* answers indicate that you saw a caring, responsive health professional.

A score of 5 to 10 *no* responses means that you may have to take the lead by asking questions and requesting information. You also may consider sending your doctor a copy of this test. He may appreciate knowing how he rated.

More than 10 *nos* mean you might want to look for another doctor. There's no reason to put up with someone who doesn't serve your needs.

8. Did the doctor discuss other possible options to the tests, treatments and/or medications you received?
Yes   No   NA
   a. If no, has the doctor *ever* discussed such options?
   Yes   No   NA

9. Did the doctor tell you about any publications or other sources of information about your condition and its control or treatment?
Yes   No   NA
   a. If no, has this doctor *ever* done so?
   Yes   No   NA

10. Were you provided with information on organizations or support groups that might be able to help you cope with your condition?
Yes   No   NA
   a. If no, has this doctor *ever* provided such information?
   Yes   No   NA

11. Was any information provided about how to prevent your condition's recurrence in the future?
Yes   No   NA
   a. If no, has this doctor *ever* provided you with such information?
   Yes   No   NA

12. Were you told about the fees prior to your visit?
Yes   No   NA

13. Were the costs of any tests, treatments and/or medications received during the visit discussed before such services were performed?
Yes   No   NA

14. If alternative tests, treatments and/or medications were discussed, did the doctor compare these costs to those of the tests, treatments and/or medications recommended?
Yes   No   NA

15. Do you consider your bill reasonable?
Yes   No   NA

16. Was it itemized in an understandable way?
Yes   No   NA

17. Did the doctor or his staff discuss what parts of your visit were covered by Medicare, Medicaid or other forms of insurance?
Yes   No   NA

18. Do you plan to use this doctor again?
Yes   No   NA

19. Would you recommend this doctor to a friend or family member?
Yes   No   NA

20. Overall, do you rate this doctor's performance as good to excellent?
Yes   No   NA

Who's Who?

Did you ever wonder just what an endocrinologist does? Have you ever confused a physiatrist with a psychiatrist? Did you know that the specialist who deals with difficult cases of arthritis is called a rheumatologist? Knowing which specialists treat what conditions can be extremely confusing to just about anyone who doesn't have a medical degree. To help, we've listed the most common types of health professionals and explained what they do and which conditions they treat. After all, if you want the best care, it helps to know which doctor to see.

A

Allergist. Diagnoses, determines the cause of and treats allergic symptoms. Uses skin tests to determine which substances provoke allergic skin reactions or hay fever. Also treats asthmatics.

Anesthesiologist. Administers the anesthetic that keeps a patient asleep during surgery. Monitors heartbeat, pulse and blood pressure during the operation. Also specializes in treating patients with respiratory failure.

Angiographer. A type of radiologist who, using catheters, injects dye into blood vessels to diagnose tumors, find bleeding sites and decide if tissue damage to blood vessels is operable. Can also stop internal bleeding by a variety of methods.

C

Cardiac Surgeon. Operates on the heart to replace diseased heart valves, remove aneurysms from the aorta and bypass blocked arteries.

Cardioangiologist. Specializes in the relationship between the heart and blood vessels.

D

Dermatologist. Diagnoses and treats diseases of the skin. Manages serious, chronic skin conditions like psoriasis and unusual rashes that fail to respond to ordinary treatment.

E

Endocrinologist. Measures hormones and treats related conditions, including difficult cases of diabetes and thyroid problems. Practices internal medicine and specializes in problems that arise from the endocrine glands such as the thyroid, pituitary, adrenals, thymus, testes and ovaries. Works with infertile couples and is called upon to interpret unusual laboratory test results.

F

Family Practitioner. Has training in medicine, pediatrics, obstetrics, gynecology and psychiatry. Cares for the family as a unit and considers their social circumstances when prescribing treatment. Usually deals with health maintenance and the prevention of disease.

G

Gastroenterologist. Specializes in diseases of the digestive organs, including the esophagus, stomach, bowel, liver and pancreas. Consulted to manage inflammatory bowel disease, chronic liver disease and problems following abdominal surgery.

General Practitioner. A primary care physician who does not limit his practice to one specialty. A G.P. can be consulted about almost any problem or symptom.

General Surgeon. Performs all types of surgery but is trained primarily in abdominal, gynecological and vascular surgery. Removes the appendix, uterus, gallbladder, polyps, moles and cysts and also repairs hernias.

Geriatrician. Specializes in the problems of aging and diseases of the elderly. Helps older persons to live happier and more satisfying lives by preventing disease and by encouraging a sound mental attitude toward aging itself.

Gynecologist. Deals with diseases of the genital tract in women and problems related to menstruation, reproduction and the pelvic organs. Performs surgery and prescribes methods of birth control.

H

Hematologist. Concerned with diseases of the blood. Treats rare anemias and other blood disorders, manages blood banks and performs bone marrow biopsies. Many also specialize in treating cancer.

I

Immunologist. Specializes in the study of immunology, that is, the way the body recognizes what is part of it (self) from what is not (nonself). Thus, an immunologist studies how the body fights off infections, responds to vaccines and reacts to allergens.

Infectious Disease Specialist. Helps hospitalized patients who have serious infections, investigates persistent fevers of uncertain origin, treats unusual infections and advises physicians on the use of potent antibiotics.

Internist. Concerned with medical (as opposed to surgical) treatment, this specialist is thoroughly trained in physical examination and diagnosis, as well as the use of sophisticated laboratory tests. Can handle complex medical problems as well as simple ones. An internist not only treats problems of the internal organs but also helps with rashes, backaches, ear, nose and throat problems, gynecology and emotional problems.

N

Neonatologist. Deals with the medical problems of newborn infants.

Nephrologist. Specializes in diseases of the kidney. Can take tissue samples of the organ through a needle, supervises dialysis procedures and works with kidney transplant cases.

Neurologist. Diagnoses and/or treats disorders of the nervous system, such as multiple sclerosis and Parkinson's disease. Consulted for unusual cases of weakness, headache, dizziness, numbness and seizures.

Neuropsychiatrist. Combines the disciplines of neurology and psychiatry to treat problems that are a combination of nervous system and mental disorders.

Neurosurgeon. An expert in surgery that relates to the nervous system. Removes brain tumors, operates on carotid arteries, removes disks and fuses the bones of the vertebrae.

Nuclear Medicine Specialist. Uses radioactive materials to diagnose problems by providing images of organs like the liver, pancreas, spleen, kidney and heart, and the bones, without resorting to surgery.

O

Obstetrician. Cares for women during pregnancy, through labor and delivery, and for a time afterward.

Oncologist. Treats patients with malignant diseases. This cancer specialist is an expert in chemotherapy and is consulted before cancer surgery is performed.

Ophthalmologist. Also known as an oculist, specializes in diagnosis and treatment of diseases and injuries of the eye, performs delicate eye surgery, such as the removal of cataracts, and is consulted whenever there is eye pain or sudden loss of vision.

Oral Surgeon. This type of dentist is most like a physician, and many actually have an M.D. Performs complex surgery on the cheek and jaw and also is called on to perform multiple tooth extractions for the elderly with medical problems.

Orthopedic Surgeon. Also known simply as an orthopedist. Sets bones, replaces diseased and damaged joints (like hips) with artificial parts and cares for patients with traumatic injuries to the skeletal system.

Osteopath. Licensed to practice medicine, prescribe drugs and perform surgery; has a D.O. (Doctor of Osteopathy) instead of an M.D. degree. Usually a generalist rather than a specialist, and differs most from M.D.'s by including manipulation as a method of treatment and diagnosis.

Otolaryngologist. Deals with ear, nose and throat disorders. Takes out tonsils and adenoids. Consulted for hearing loss, ear infections, sinusitis, long-term hoarseness and persistent nosebleeds.

P

Pathologist. Known for determining the exact cause of death by performing an autopsy. Also an expert in identifying disease-related changes in the body's tissues and organs, determining whether a tissue sample is benign or malignant.

Pediatrician. Specializes in the medical care of children, especially those under 3 and those with serious childhood diseases. Some pediatricians also subspecialize in a specific area of medicine, such as pediatric neurosurgery or pediatric cardiology.

Physiatrist. Specializes in physical medicine and rehabilitation. Combines orthopedics, neurology, classical medicine and physical therapy to restore sick or disabled patients to their best level of functioning.

Plastic Surgeon. "Cosmetic" surgery ranges from performing facelifts and "nose jobs" to restoring the appearance and function of the skin of burn patients, facial reconstructing of victims of disfiguring accidents and correcting birth defects like cleft palate. Cosmetic or reconstructive surgery requires a deft and delicate hand to perform relatively scar-free work.

Proctologist. Concerned with disorders of the rectum and the anus. Consulted for hemorrhoids, rectal bleeding, anal exams and surgery.

Psychiatrist. Deals with the study, treatment and prevention of mental illness. Trained in diagnosis and therapy. Also may investigate possible organic causes for mental illness and prescribe drugs.

Pulmonary Specialist. Deals with people on respirators, diagnoses unusual lung disorders and works with people who have chronic lung diseases or asthma. Consulted in cases of extreme shortness of breath.

R

Radiologist. Specializes in taking and interpreting X rays, as well as in using X ray technology and other diagnostic aids, like ultrasound and CAT scans, to diagnose physical problems.

Rheumatologist. Deals with problems and diseases of the joints and connective tissue, manages diseases like rheumatoid arthritis, SLE (lupus) and scleroderma. Consulted on questions relating to arthritis treatment and musculoskeletal problems.

S

Surgeon. See *General Surgeon*. There are also some surgeons who specialize in specific areas such as abdominal, rectal, thoracic, endocrine, cardiac and vascular surgery.

T

Thoracic Surgeon. Handles surgery that involves opening up the chest cavity, including procedures on the lungs, heart and major blood vessels.

U

Urologist. Deals with problems of the bladder and surgical problems involving the kidney. Treats urinary tract infections and problems of the penis, scrotum and prostate.

V

Vascular Surgeon. Operates on the arteries, bypassing blocked arteries and removing the fatty material that narrows the artery, especially in the lower heart and in the legs.

What's What

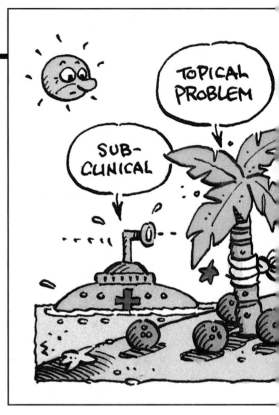

The cartoons to the right are meant to give a little giggle, but the humor stops when a physician explains something to you in "doctorspeak" instead of plain English. You may think, for example, you're failing math if the doctor explains that you have a problem with calculus. What he means, of course, is there's a stone in your kidney or gallbladder. Similarly, a clavicle isn't the physician's favorite musical instrument but rather the medical term for your collarbone. Subclinical does not mean that you should go to the hospital's basement but that your problem is very mild. And a topical medicine is applied to the surface of your body, not where the palm trees sway.

As you can see, it's helpful for you to become familiar with some commonly used medical terms. Take this little quiz and see how many of them you know the meaning of—without a dictionary.

1. Does *adipose* mean: (a) fatty tissue; (b) a reclining position; (c) the person who totals your hospital bill.
Answer: (*a*). The more overweight you are, the more adipose tissue there is in your body.

2. If you're *ambulatory,* that means: (a) you have to ride in the ambulance; (b) you can walk on your own; (c) you are able to walk no farther than the bathroom.
Answer: (*b*). Just think of being able to amble about.

3. If your doctor thinks you need a mild *analgesic,* he wants you to take: (a) a painkiller; (b) rectal medicine; (c) a tranquilizer.
Answer: (*a*). Despite the fact that it starts with *anal-,* an analgesic is a pain reliever, such as aspirin. The prefix *an-* means "no," and the *-algesic* part of the word stands for "pain."

4. If your doctor thinks you should be taking an *antipyretic* medicine, he wants to: (a) relieve your itching; (b) help your burning, upset stomach; (c) reduce your fever.
Answer: (*c*). The beginning of the word, *anti-,* means "against," of course, and *-pyr* means "fire," as in *pyromaniac.* So an antipyretic works against the fires raging inside your body.

5. If a doctor wants to discuss *atrophy,* he intends to talk about: (a) a traditional hospital award for best patient; (b) helping you lose weight carefully; (c) shrinkage of muscles or other tissue.

Answer: (*c*). When you wear a cast, for instance, the muscles underneath shrink up from lack of use. Luckily, that kind of atrophy is temporary and the muscles will regain their original size and strength. Atrophy can also be a symptom of more serious disorders.

6. If you are told that the growth your doctor removed was *benign,* that means: (a) it was not cancerous; (b) it *was* found to be cancerous; (c) it was growing very quickly.
Answer: (*a*). Benign means good news—no cancerous cells were found. A *malignant* growth is cancerous.

7. A *congenital* condition is one that: (a) is inherited; (b) affects the genital area; (c) was present at birth.
Answer: (*c*). These conditions, such as congenital heart defects, develop before you are even born.

8. If something is *contraindicated,* you should: (a) take it; (b) avoid it; (c) take it every other day.
Answer: (*b*). Aspirin, for instance, is contraindicated for people with stomach ulcers, because it can cause additional internal bleeding.

9. If you have *dermatitis,* it means your skin is: (a) too tight; (b) inflamed; (c) numb.
Answer: (*b*). When a word ends in *-itis,* it means "inflammation." With dermatitis, there may be itching, rash, redness and inflammation.

10. The word *edema* means: (a) swelling; (b) bruising; (c) lack of intelligence.
Answer: (*a*). When body tissues hold an excessive

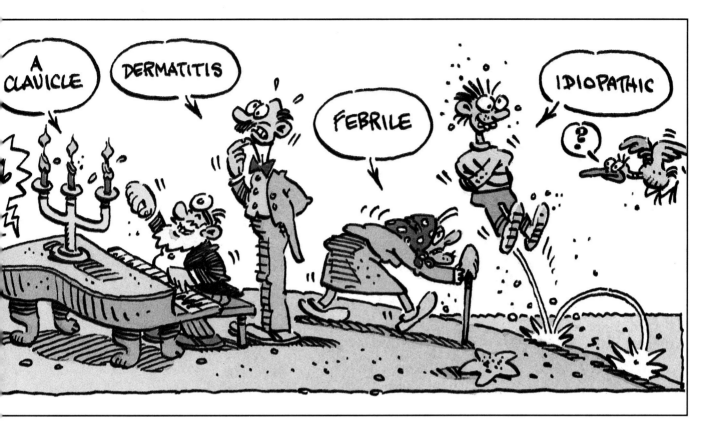

amount of fluid, the area swells up. It is common to see edema in the ankles and feet of pregnant women. But it could also be a sign of a problem with kidney function.

11. *Etiology* refers to: (a) the study of food and nutrition; (b) the cause of an illness or disease; (c) hospital or medical etiquette.
Answer: (*b*). It's a sophisticated way of discussing the cause of a medical problem.

12. If your doctor says that you're *febrile*, he's saying that you are: (a) old and weak; (b) feverish; (c) in need of more dietary fiber.
Answer: (*b*). Someone in a febrile state may also feel weak, but they definitely have a fever.

13. A *hematoma* is: (a) a bruise; (b) a medical instrument; (c) a disease only men get.
Answer: (*a*). The word refers to a bruise anywhere on your body.

14. A *hemorrhage* means: (a) massive blood loss; (b) any blood loss; (c) loss of a particular type of blood.
Answer: (*b*). Although we mostly hear about serious hemorrhaging, this term refers to any kind of bleeding.

15. *Idiopathic* means: (a) lower intelligence; (b) a malignant area of the body; (c) of unknown cause.
Answer: (*c*). When a doctor uses this word in referring to a disease or condition, it means he doesn't know what's causing the problem.

16. A *lesion* is: (a) any kind of sore or wound; (b) a group of military doctors; (c) a surgical procedure.
Answer: (*a*). It's a very broad term that includes wounds, sores, ulcers and any other tissue damage.

17. If your test results are *negative*, it means: (a) you do have the problem; (b) you don't have the problem; (c) your condition is critical.
Answer: (*b*). A negative result is *good* news, because it means you don't have the problem or disorder they were testing you for.

18. *Parenteral* refers to: (a) the health of your mother or father; (b) a disease inherited from your parents; (c) a way to administer medication.
Answer: (*c*). Instead of "Mom and Dad," the word means "not by mouth," indicating that the medicine is to be injected and not taken in oral form.

19. If you have a condition accompanied by *pruritus*, one of your problems is: (a) pus forming around the wound; (b) itching; (c) an allergy to cats.
Answer: (*b*). An itch by any other name should still probably not be scratched.

20. The word *sequela* refers to: (a) being kept in quarantine; (b) an extremely quiet atmosphere; (c) the aftereffects of a disease.
Answer: (*c*). Just think of the word sequel and you've got the answer. A sequela occurs when one disorder develops as a result of another.

Doctoring from Nondoctors

Nurse Practitioner (N.P.)—To become an N.P., a nurse must study for an additional year. This health professional is qualified to handle routine medical problems like colds and earaches under a physician's supervision. A medical doctor is called upon to treat more serious conditions.

Optometrist—After 4 years of study at a school of optometry, this practitioner performs complete eye exams and prescribes corrective lenses, but can't treat eye problems or disorders.

Chiropractic Doctor (D.C.)—Not licensed to prescribe drugs or perform surgery, chiropractors manipulate the spine and use other physical therapies.

Podiatrist (D.P.M.)—Formerly known as chiropodists, podiatrists attend a podiatric medical school for 4 years. They can prescribe medications, perform surgery and treat all conditions pertaining to the feet.

Clinical Psychologist—After receiving a Ph.D. from an accredited university, these professionals function as therapists who treat people with emotional difficulties. They cannot prescribe drugs.

Dentist (D.D.S. or D.M.D.)—This degree requires 4 years of study at a dental college. A dentist writes prescriptions, fills, pulls, straightens and caps teeth. Specialization requires 5 additional years of classroom and practical experience.

Physical Therapist—Having completed a course of study in an approved school of physical therapy, these professionals use exercise and other physical means to relieve pain and improve muscular function.

Certified Nurse-Midwife (C.N.M.)—These are registered nurses with specialized education in obstetrics. They deliver babies with a minimum of medical intervention and provide prenatal and postnatal care.

EXAMINING THE EXAMINATION

"A good doctor works hard," when he gives you a physical, says Dr. LeMaitre, who offers this checklist as "an excellent test of your doctor's thoroughness."

Your doctor should check:

- Vital signs, including your blood pressure (preferably in *both* arms, for comparison), pulse, respiration and temperature.
- Your skin, head, ears, nose, throat, mouth, neck, chest, genital area and extremities.
- Your eyes, which should be tested for glaucoma and examined in a darkened room to detect the possibility of diabetes or high blood pressure.
- Your abdomen and your back, looking for tender spots over your kidneys and checking the shape and alignment of your spine.
- For women, your breasts, as well as the armpits and the depressions above the collarbone on both sides.
- Your rectum and, for men, the prostate gland.

With few exceptions, anything less than a thorough examination is a sign that something is wrong, according to Dr. LeMaitre. "Beware of the doctor who listens briefly to your chief complaint, asks very few questions, performs a rather cursory examination of the area of your complaint, prescribes a simple medication, pats you on the shoulder, reassures you and tells you to come back in a week. You've wasted your time and your money and risked your health."

DON'T SPECIALIZE WHEN YOU CAN GENERALIZE

Should you discover that your present doctor is less than ideal and decide to look for a new one, here's how doctors themselves suggest that you begin your search.

"Your best source for finding a physician is the closest medical center or medical school," says Lila A. Wallis, M.D., clinical professor of medicine at Cornell University Medical College in New York City. "In a teaching institution, the students' questions keep the doctors current — and honest."

If you're unsure which are "teaching hospitals" and which aren't, just call up and ask if the local hospital in question is a teaching institution and which university or medical school it is affiliated with. You can also do the reverse — check your phone book for medical schools, call the closest ones and ask for the name of their hospital.

Another way to find a doctor suited to you is to call your county medical society. Although their referrals will not have been well screened, Dr. Wallis feels that they are an excellent source for finding young doctors who are just starting up a practice in your area.

Dr. Wallis feels that these young doctors, who have joined the medical society to find new patients, will be eager to please. There is a better chance, she feels, that they will make house calls and be available in emergencies.

Perhaps you're a woman who's had it with male doctors who patronize you, or you think that women M.D.'s tend to be a little more caring and human. If so, some local branches of the American Medical Women's Association (AMWA) will provide a list of physicians in your area.

"Patients who feel they need a lot of explanations and who wish to be partners in their own health care may do better with a woman physician," feels Dr. Wallis. "As a general rule, women tend to spend more time with patients. They may be more willing to teach, to explain, to communicate."

No matter whom you call for a recommendation, Dr. Wallis suggests that you ask for three different names and urges that you specify whether you want a family practitioner or an internist.

Those titles are important — you want to avoid the medical mistake of having a specialist for your everyday health care. As an example, Dr. Wallis notes that, "80 to 85 percent of women are using a gynecologist as their primary physician — and that's a mistake.

"The woman with a gynecologist as her primary care physician thinks of herself as existing only below the waist. She needs someone skilled in listening to the heart, performing breast exams and thyroid exams and checking blood pressure. Many good gynecologists *do* extend the scope of their skills in these areas, but most have the training and outlook of surgeons," notes Dr. Wallis, "and are therefore *not* the doctors for everyday problems."

TEST-DRIVE THAT NEW DOCTOR

You've narrowed your search down to the right kind of doctor and you've gotten the names of likely prospects. Now, how do you make that final choice?

"It's important that the prospective patient not try to interview the doctor on the phone," says Dr. Wallis. Instead, she suggests a long talk with the office secretary.

"Ask what to expect on the first visit. Will the doctor order any tests, and what will it all cost? Is there anything that you as the patient should bring with you?

"Family history is extremely important," says Dr. Wallis, "as is your own medical history. If you arrive with most of those details, including dates and duration of illnesses and medications, already written down, it will save a lot of time normally spent on paperwork. That leaves more time for a good exam and for you to get to know the doctor better."

That personal contact — the feeling that you and your doctor establish with each other — is the key to finding the right doctor for you.

"Paper certification does not produce professional excellence," points out Dr. LeMaitre. "No matter how many degrees a doctor has, how many pieces of paper claiming expertise in this or that branch of medicine, performance is what counts.

"Heart," he says. "That is what separates the excellent physician from the mediocre."

8

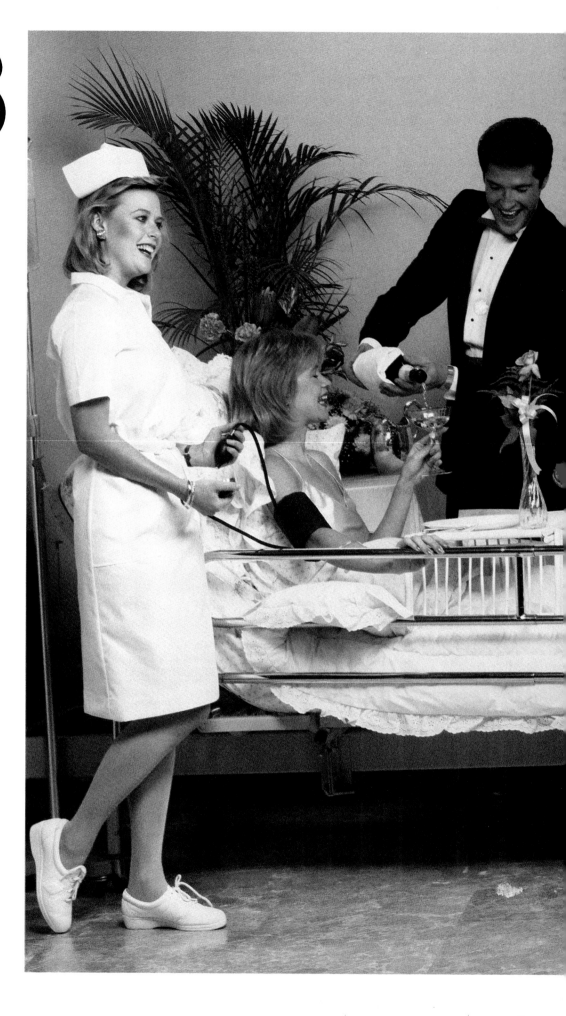

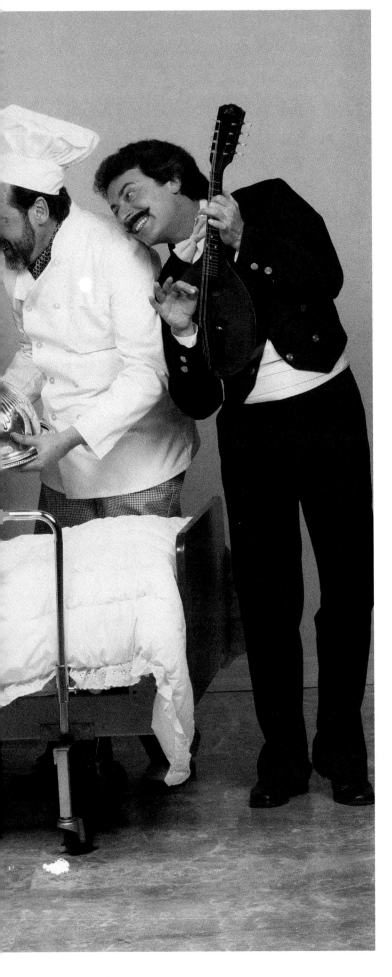

Making Hospitals Work for You

Knowledge is power and leads to successful and cost-effective health care.

When Princess Grace failed to negotiate a hairpin turn and plunged her car down a steep French mountainside, the choice of hospitals became a matter of life and death.

Unfortunately, she was rushed to a small facility in her home principality of Monaco instead of a larger, more technologically advanced hospital in Paris or Nice. The hospital didn't even have CAT scan equipment to diagnose her severe head injury. As precious moments slipped by, French neurologists had to be located and flown in. And when they arrived, they were too late. The curtains had been drawn over the life of the former actress.

A number of doctors in France and America were quoted as saying the Princess could have been saved had she been taken to the right hospital.

And when hospital and state inspectors failed to detect crossed oxygen and anesthetic lines in a Pennsylvania hospital, five people were killed when they were administered nitrous oxide instead of lifesaving oxygen. The mixed lines remained undetected for *seven months!*

One could conclude from these two incidents that choosing the wrong hospital is deadly. However, that conclusion probably would be wrong. These extreme cases should by no means indict the entire world hospital system. Today's hospitals are places where the human body can be repaired in ways that were only the wild fantasies of science fiction writers a decade ago. Brilliant researchers have teamed with precision technology to devise treatments for scores of once-incurable illnesses.

What they have yet to cure are mistakes and spiraling costs. The best surgeons and most wondrous machines are costly, and they will never eliminate the need to be careful.

You can cut both risks and expenses by educating yourself about what's good, bad and costly in today's hospitals.

HOSPITAL TAKEOVERS

Imagine a giant PacMan with a voracious appetite for hospitals. That image could represent the current revolution in hospitals. The PacMen are huge conglomerates like the Hospital Corporation of America (HCA), based in Nashville, Tennessee, and Humana, Inc., of Louisville, Kentucky, and they're taking over nonbusiness hospitals and turning them into profit-making enterprises. At last count, HCA, the largest conglomerate, owns and operates 450 hospitals in 46 states and eight foreign countries.

What does this mean to you, the patient?

That question has raged for a decade with no answer in sight. James E. Bryan, formerly the executive director of the New York County Medical Society, believes big business has no business in the medical profession.

"Medicine is changing, from a patient-centered caring universe of community-oriented hospitals singularly devoted to prolonging and enriching human life, into an industry offering the affluent few an opportunity to draw handsome profits from the sicknesses and misfortunes of the many," Bryan charges in an article in the *Washington Post*.

"It is the ultimate naiveté to expect a hospital to act like a local community service when it is owned by a remote, profit-seeking corporation whose components are all lashed to the bottom line. Will you be able to call him or her 'your doctor' when he examines you courtesy of U.S. Medicine, Inc?" Bryan continues.

Sure you will, counter the conglomerates. They argue that Bryan's statements reflect old fears that have failed to materialize. David Rollo, M.D., Ph.D., senior vice president of medical affairs for Humana, Inc., says the group-owned system enables hospitals to make mass purchases of supplies and equipment while allowing them to establish quality standards, to have greater access to medical information and to share technology, skills and advances among the chain hospitals. As for impersonal service, Dr. Rollo sharply disagrees.

"It's quite the contrary. We have an educational program, called Humanacare, which teaches our doctors and staff the art of caring, listening, being empathic and responding to the needs of the patients. Humana has found this program to be very effective," he says.

Until enough studies are made to settle the issue, Charles B. Inlander, executive director of the People's Medical Society (PMS), suggests keeping close tabs on your area corporate-owned hospital. Be on the lookout for rising costs, overspecialization and a total shut-out of poor and uninsured patients.

"Let your voice be heard," Inlander says. "If your hospital has boards that include citizen members, try to get on them. Bring attention to unsatisfactory situations or conditions. Write letters to the editor, call television and radio stations. If so moved, organize and lead protests against offending institutions. Urge politicians to concern themselves with the health and medical interests of their constituents."

PICKING A WINNER

All things considered, the owner of your local hospital may not be as important as its staff. Hospital care still depends, as Bryan says, on the "human factors—the doctors, nurses and health professionals." In chapter 7, you learned how to select a good doctor. Thomas O'Donovan, Ph.D., president of the American Academy of Medical Administrators, says that this selection is also the single most important factor in choosing a hospital. And he discounts critics who say doctors just refer you to the hospital that offers them privileges.

"Good doctors don't select bad hospitals," Dr. O'Donovan says. "In the case of major surgery or specialized care, your doctor knows the best place for the care you need. If it's not

What We Know about

HMO

John Doe   Expires ⁶/₈₉

On Wall Street, they see it strictly in financial terms. The health insurance industry is embroiled in a blistering battle as reigning champion Blue Cross/Blue Shield is being challenged by a powerful new contender— the Health Maintenance Organization (HMO). Unless you invest in insurance stocks, all you really need to know is: Which gives the best care?

There's no real cut-and-dried answer. An HMO may be great for you but not so great for your neighbor. Here's how HMOs work, along with some positives and negatives.

HMOs differ from Blue Cross/Blue Shield and most traditional medical plans in that they are a subscriber service; that is, an employer prepays a fixed amount for an employee health benefit program. Instead of picking your own doctor, however, you choose a doctor from a list of available HMO doctors. This person is now your "assigned" doctor. He will refer you to HMO-affiliated specialists if further care is needed. The fees for office visits are minimal, usually $2, with the specialists covered completely by the plan.

"The best thing about HMOs is that they provide incentive to keep the population well," says Lowell S. Levin, Ed.D., M.P.H., of Yale University. "The less the prepaid services are used, the lower the HMO's cost of operation. To accomplish this, HMOs frequently offer free preventive health activities like exercise programs and programs that help you stop smoking.

"Since they are basically a group practice, they offer the benefit of shared knowledge among doctors. This leads to better quality control. In addition, your records are kept in one place, which streamlines communication among the health-care providers," he says.

"Another advantage is the fixed cost factor. No matter what happens, you are completely covered for nothing more than the price of a $2 office visit.

"The negatives are that you might want to go to a doctor or specialist who is not a member of the HMO group," explains Dr. Levin. "This situation is common among women who have already established a relationship with a gynecologist."

Other negatives include:

- Emergency care—An HMO doctor will be available, but he may not be the one you are used to seeing. (Such is the case, however, with much emergency care.)
- Waiting—Some HMOs may have 1- to 2-month waits for nonurgent appointments such as physical examinations.

"Before you sign up for an HMO, visit their headquarters and talk to the doctors," Dr. Levin advises. "Are they warm and attentive, or detached and bureaucratic? Is the facility clean and comfortable? Do they operate 24 hours a day, including a telephone emergency advice service? Do they have a patient advocate or some recourse system if you are unhappy with your care?

"Make sure they answer all your questions before you join," he cautions.

his hospital, he'll refer you to a specialist at another one. Trust him."

If you are new to an area, Dr. O'Donovan suggests finding a family physician or general practitioner and letting him advise you on the best local hospital.

Richard C. Inskip, M.D., president of the American Academy of Family Physicians, agrees.

"First and foremost, we do what's in the patient's best interest. We consider what services or specialties are required and refer the patient to a hospital that can provide those services," he says.

If, for some reason, you need a hospital before you settle in with a doctor, here's what you should do.

"Ask your neighbors, the people you work with, friends, or even your insurance representative to recommend a hospital," Dr. O'Donovan advises. "What you shouldn't do is look in the Yellow Pages and pick the one that's closest."

If you are confused by the different types of hospitals—small, large, general, specialized, medical centers, university-affiliated teaching hospitals, nonprofit, for-profit, etc.—Dr. Inskip and Dr. O'Donovan say the burden of choice belongs to your doctor.

"If you have a very serious heart problem and need extensive surgery, you wouldn't go to a small general hospital with a limited program," Dr. O'Donovan says. "You would go to a hospital that specializes in the heart. The same goes for any serious ailment or major surgery. But again, your doctor knows this. He'll place you where you can get the best care."

CHECKING THEM OUT

All this doesn't mean you should just go wherever your doctor points. Once he or she has made the choice, you should double-check the selection.

A good way to start is to call the hospital and find out if it has an effective in-hospital infection surveillance and control program. (Most hospitals have these programs, which keep track of and try to control infections that occur among hospital patients, but in some places the programs are second-rate and infections are still far too common.) A multiagency study headed by the U.S. Centers for Disease Control estimated that two million patients per year acquire hospital-bred infections. A companion study revealed that hospitals with good infection surveillance and control programs were able to *reduce* their infection rates by 32 percent, while hospitals without such programs suffer an *increased* infection rate of 18 percent.

To make sure the hospital is up to snuff, ask if there's a doctor on staff who's been trained in infection control, as well as one full-time infection-control nurse for every 250 beds, and if the infection-control system is computerized. If these requirements aren't met, says Robert W. Haley, M.D., author of *Managing Hospital Infection Control for Cost-Effectiveness*, then the system probably doesn't work—and you're more likely to be a victim of a bug you didn't have when you were admitted.

The next question you should ask is if the hospital employs a patient advocate or ombudsman. A person in this position is a troubleshooter whose sole function is to serve the patient by taking care of problems. Their power and exact functions vary. But the growing trend among hospital administrators is to give them enough authority to effectively solve patient dilemmas.

Medicinal Laughter

One of *Reader's Digest's* most popular features is a section titled "Laughter is the Best Medicine." Some hospitals are taking that literally and establishing "humor rooms" to add some levity to the frequently somber hospital environment. Humor rooms are playrooms for grown-ups where patients can compete in games, solve puzzles, watch upbeat movies or simply visit relatives in a cheerful atmosphere. "For 80 years scientists have looked at negative emotions—depression, hostility, anger—and their effects on health. Now we are looking at the flip side," says Deborah Leiber, R.N., founder of the 600-member Nurses for Laughter organization.

Alexandra Gekas, director of the National Society of Patient Representatives of the American Hospital Association, says 52 percent of America's 6,000 hospitals now have patient reps.

"We will do almost anything to make someone's stay as productive and comfortable as possible," Ms. Gekas explains. "We'll get more information on their illness, explain an upcoming procedure, change a room or bring their doctor back to answer questions. Whatever the patients' problems are, they shouldn't hesitate to call us."

In a similar vein, ask if the hospital staff regularly attends patient-relations programs. These are educational seminars designed to improve the attention doctors, nurses and hospital staffs pay to the human and emotional needs of the patients. If the hospital does have such a program, ask if attendance is mandatory or voluntary. If it's voluntary, ask what percentage of doctors, nurses and staff actually attend.

Also inquire about support groups. According to one survey, more than half of American hospitals operate or participate in support group programs that enable patients and former patients to share their feelings, fears and tips on how to cope with chronic disease and other stressful problems. These groups offer help to those with cancer, heart disease, alcoholism and other major afflictions.

Some additional tips:

- Trust a nurse. The lifeblood of every hospital, nurses tend to be refreshingly honest and loaded with spunk. In a study of 12,500 nurses, 83 percent said they would advise patients of non-surgical alternatives to their problems even if the doctor refused, and would do so at the risk of their jobs. In addition, because the demand for nurses is so high, they have little problem moving from job to job. As a result, they usually have an excellent grasp of which area hospitals are good and which are duds. If you know a nurse, ask for the lowdown.

- Ask questions: The People's Medical Society, the nation's largest consumer-activist group, suggests grilling the hospital admissions officer with the following:

How much will it cost? Everything, including doctor's fees, hospital costs, consulting doctors and extras. Will they accept your insurance? Once you have a dollar figure, shop around for the best hospital at the best price.

How many nurses are on staff? Look for patient/nurse ratios no greater than 4 to 1, and 2 to 1 in intensive care.

What is the secondary infection rate among surgical patients?

How many surgical procedures of the nature you require does the hospital perform each year?

- Take a walking tour to assess the cleanliness of the hospital. Are the floors clean? How does the place smell? Are the uniforms of housekeepers, orderlies and security guards clean? Are the rooms clean?

- Ask yourself and your doctor, "Do I really need to be in a hospital? If so, how soon can I get out?"

INHOSPITABLE STAYS

As conscientious as hospitals try to be, sometimes they just blow it. For the most part, their mistakes are confined to billing and accounting. Occasionally, however, the errors involve patient care and the results are tragic. Studies have pinned down some of the most frequent mistakes. Public awareness will help keep them from recurring.

A study by Walter E. Stamm, M.D., done at the University of Washington School of Medicine, concluded that 850,000 hospitalized patients per year are infected by the medical devices used to treat them. The riskiest devices were urinary catheters, intravenous infusion devices, hemodialysis equipment and respiratory therapy equipment. Dr. Stamm recommended tighter controls, including catheter care teams, aseptic insertion, more frequent catheter changes, closer bacteriologic mon-

Club "Med"

It's not so much Club Med as Club Medical, but even so, weekend retreats geared for the elderly at area hospitals are becoming the rage. North Penn Hospital in Lansdale, Pennsylvania, started it when they offered $179 getaway weekend packages that combined fun, food and recreation with nursing care. It was designed to give a breather to those caring for sick, elderly relatives as well as to help the patients themselves. It became such a hit North Penn officials are now teaching other hospitals to do the same.

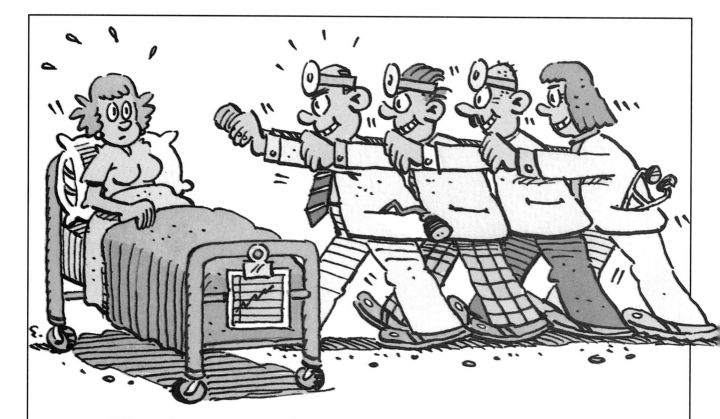

Must Strangers with Stethoscopes Examine You?

You have an illness or injury. You've been hospitalized by your doctor so he can keep an eye on it. But soon a lot of eyes are involved. A parade of doctors, nurses, technicians, interns, residents and medical students comes in and takes a peek. Any moment you expect the maid to mosey over and lift the sheets. You've done more strip-tease acts than Gypsy Rose Lee! What gives?

You. Your silence has given them carte blanche to use your body as a medical experiment. Speak up. You have the right to refuse examination by any-

one, M.D.'s included, who don't have your explicit permission. An examination by someone without your consent may constitute unauthorized touching and could provide the basis for a lawsuit. Discuss the issue with your doctor. But before you decree hands off, consider that doctors often have associates double-check their patients to offer suggestions and confirm the original diagnosis. This works in your favor. And the interns, residents and medical students have to learn. One of them may be your next doctor.

itoring, better training among those who administer the devices, stronger manufacturer concern and other safety procedures. If you are about to be treated with any of these devices, ask your doctor what precautions are taken to ensure you won't be infected.

In another study of hospital patients, this one headed by Knight Steel, M.D., and Paul M. Gertman,

M.D., and conducted at the Boston University Medical Center, 815 people were surveyed. It was found that 36 percent of them had developed an illness not related in any way to the condition for which they were hospitalized—an illness related instead to the hospital stay itself. Nine percent of the illnesses were life-threatening or produced disability, while 2 percent contributed to a patient's death. The specific causes, ranging from therapeutic procedures to transportation and nursing errors, are too diverse to list here. However, one factor—drug side effects—was significant.

"Exposure to drugs seems to be a particularly important factor in determining which patients have complications, and such exposure was also associated with increased severity of complications," say the researchers.

While the researchers focused their recommendations on precautions to be implemented by doctors, hospital administrators and other health professionals, the patient also can play a role. When the nurse hands you the little pleated paper cup containing medicine, demand to know what that drug *is*, as well as its possible side effects or interactions with other drugs or foods. Be on guard.

Other hospital hazards to beware of include:

Electrical Shock. A study headed by Sidney R. Arbeit, M.D., and conducted at the Montefiore Hospital and Medical Center in the Bronx, found hospital patients could be subject to electrical shock due to poorly designed electrical devices and inadequate or improper grounding of the hospital electrical system or equipment. The study recommended modernizing the building wiring, employing better grounding techniques, performing more safety checks of new equipment and establishing an electrical preventive maintenance program.

Malnutrition. A real irony is that some hospital food not only tastes bad, it's also nutritionally bankrupt! After a rash of stories and studies detailing this in the past decade, many hospitals have established nutritional support units. Check to see if your hospital has one.

EMERGENCY CARE

It's Thanksgiving day. You're flinging a Frisbee with the kids. Suddenly, you feel as though Mr. T has jumped

---

Hospital Procedures You Don't Need

"Shave the whole belly," the doctor barks before entering the operating room. The patient, cold and exposed, must go under the blade as well as the knife—and afterward suffer the itch of regrowth along with the pinch of healing.

Recent evidence has shown that the shaving isn't always warranted. A British study determined that patients shaved prior to abdominal surgery, a common technique thought to lessen postoperative infection, had a higher infection rate than those left unshaved.

In addition, hospitals sometimes submit patients to procedures that do little but hurt, jumble your emotions and deplete your finances.

Checking in? Slide up to the cold X ray machine for a dose of radiation. Then bring your arm (and wallet) over to the vampires in the blood lab. Having a baby? Expect an enema during labor.

Well, maybe not. The American College of Radiology has recommended that chest X rays no longer be included in routine hospital admission procedures because of the minuscule number of diseases detected in that manner. University of California researchers have denounced routine preoperative blood tests for similar reasons.

As for the enemas, another British study of 274 pregnant women contradicted the common belief that an anal wash lowers the chance of fecal contamination and infection during delivery and makes labor less difficult. The study found enemas made *no* difference in infection or labor. And neither does the scratchy shave.

---

on your chest. You suspect a heart attack and realize you need immediate emergency care. But where should you go? The closest hospital is 30 minutes away. Then you remember the new emergency center in the mall up the street. The 20 minutes you save might mean life or death. What do you do?

"First of all, you shouldn't be making a decision like that after the emergency strikes," admonishes Dr. Inskip. "You should have already planned where you will go in an emergency before it happens."

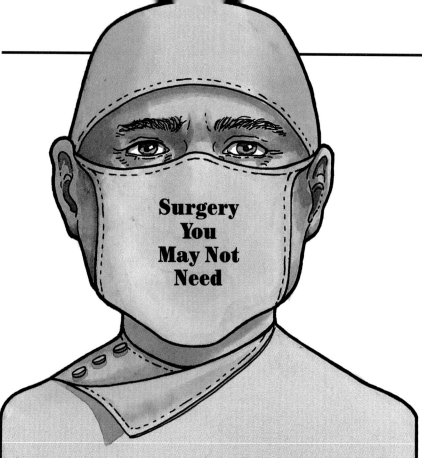

Surgery You May Not Need

Accusations have swirled in the past decade over the possibility that many surgeons are too quick with the knife. Heart specialist Robert G. Schneider, M.D., estimates that 15 to 25 percent of all operations are unnecessary, which means 3 to 6 million unneeded operations are performed each year. *RN* magazine polled 12,500 nurses and discovered that 46 percent placed the unnecessary surgery figure at 30 percent or higher.

A statistical review by the authors of *Take This Book to the Hospital with You* has zeroed in on part of the problem. As surgeons flood the market, say authors Charles B. Inlander and Ed Weiner, the number of operations has increased. While the population is growing at only 5 percent a year, the rate of operations leaps up 35 percent annually.

Furthermore, they have identified some specific types of surgery that appear to be overdone. They are mastectomies, hysterectomies, cesarean sections, tonsillectomies and breast biopsies.

Of course, not all operations in these categories are unwarranted, but some may be. If you are scheduled for one of these procedures, get a second and even a third opinion. For additional help, consult either Dr. Schneider's book *When to Say No to Surgery,* or *The Prevention Guide to Surgery and Its Alternatives.*

Dr. Inskip says this preparation is even more vital if you are considering going to a freestanding emergency clinic.

"You have to carefully evaluate whether these so-called Docs in the Box or Mall Medicine clinics can handle a true emergency. Some have the capabilities to handle life-and-death situations like heart attacks, while others don't," says Dr. Inskip. "Many are just ambulatory care centers. What you should do is ask your family physician what he knows about the facility. What kind of equipment do they have? Are doctors available 24 hours? Is the place open for 24 hours? Is it open on holidays?"

Judith Ryan, R.N., Ph.D., executive director of the American Nurses' Association, agrees that you should check out the emergency clinic the moment it comes to your neighborhood.

"I would be very careful as a consumer. The problem with many of these freestanding clinics is that they specialize in only one service, like weight loss, nutrition, cancer care or general practice. They may not have the emergency capabilities you need. Check with your local nurses' association, which should be listed under 'Associations' in the Yellow Pages. They should be able to explain the benefits and flaws of local emergency clinics."

HOSPITAL EMERGENCY ROOMS

If you haven't checked out the local clinic, you'd better call an ambulance to take you to the hospital.

"Again, the bottom line is, you should know where to go *before* the emergency," Dr. Inskip emphasizes. "You should have a personal physician whom you can reach on a 24-hour basis. If you describe your symptoms, your doctor will tell you what to do and where to go. Often he'll tell you that you don't need to do anything more than come to the office in the morning."

Bruce Janiak, M.D., director of the emergency center at Toledo Hospital in Ohio, offers these additional pointers.

- Find out what hospital your doctor recommends before an emergency. Generally it will be the one he uses, and going there will help with record-keeping.
- Post emergency phone numbers (including an ambulance service) alongside your telephone.
- Keep written first-aid tips handy. If someone in your family has a heart problem, Dr. Janiak says the rest of the family should be trained in cardiopulmonary resuscitation.
- Know what your local emergency services are and how to use them. Many hospital or private ambulance companies are now staffed with emergency medical technicians or paramedics. They can begin your care before you get to the hospital.

June Thompson, R.N., an assistant professor at the University of Texas Health Science Center, Houston, says there are six questions you should ask when scouting for an emergency room. These can apply to hospital services or freestanding clinics.

- Are the doctors and nurses certified in emergency care? "There are now board-certified emergency physicians and a certification program for emergency nurses," Ms. Thompson explains.
- What kind of emergency department is it? Some are trauma centers staffed around the clock with doctors and nurses trained to handle serious injuries. Surgical facilities are immediately available. Other emergency rooms (ERs) are staffed by family physicians, interns or moonlighting doctors. Some ERs operate by having physicians on call, meaning they have to track down the doctor. "I might go to one hospital if I were sick, and another, the trauma center, if I were injured," Ms. Thompson says.
- If you call an ambulance, can you decide which hospital to go to? It's possible, but it probably is best to let the ambulance crew decide. They know which hospital is best for your problem.
- Will a nurse or doctor examine you within five minutes after

Cutting Surgery Costs

If you must go under the knife, here are some ways to avoid a "walletectomy."

1. Find out if you can have the operation on an outpatient basis.

2. Get a second opinion on elective surgery and call your insurance company to see if it is covered.

3. Ask the surgeon what his fee will be and what it will include.

4. Ask if preoperative and postoperative visits are included in the fee.

5. Find out if any assistants will be in on the operation and if you will be charged for them.

6. Ask what your family doctor will charge if he visits you in the hospital.

7. Make sure you know when you can go home, and go.

8. Keep all personal supplies that have been charged to you.

9. Ask the surgeon if he knows of any aspect of the operation your insurance won't cover.

10. If you are given medical trinkets such as cotton balls or ointments upon discharge, say, "no thanks." You may be charged a markup over drugstore prices.

you arrive? "They should take vital signs and determine your medical history," says Ms. Thompson. "That doesn't mean you'll be treated right away, but

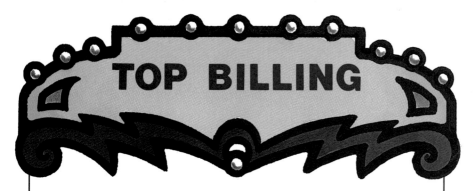

TOP BILLING

How expensive can a hospital stay be? A hospital in Houston, Texas, billed Marine Engineers Beneficial Association of Baltimore, Maryland, $447,574 for a patient's 5-month stay. That comes to $2,500 a day. A hospital in Boston billed the same insurer $238,000 for a subscriber's 37-day stay. That came to a whopping $6,525 per day, 38 times the national average. Needless to say, the insurance company is investigating.

know some basic truths about hospitals and their billing systems. According to the People's Medical Society:

- Mathematical mistakes often go undetected.
- You are frequently billed for things you don't need or want, or never received.
- You are charged for a gauntlet of expensive, unnecessary tests.
- The markup charged for drugs, vitamins, plastic trays and other items is often extremely high.
- Rates for identical services can vary tremendously from hospital to hospital.

The key to avoiding the white-coat rip-off is to go over your bill with a fine-tooth comb (yours, not one they supply).

"Don't sign anything and don't give your approval to anything until you are satisfied that your bill is entirely correct," advises Charles Inlander of PMS. "Ask questions about anything that isn't clear or seems odd to you. If costs can't be justified, have them eliminated. If the bill is riddled with inaccuracies, don't pay it. Talk to the head of the department to have it corrected.

"If the bill is too long to examine in the cashier's office, take it home. Then bring it back to the hospital and settle up. The hospital cannot stop you from leaving," Inlander says.

Before going to the hospital, check with your doctor to find out what tests will be done and if they are necessary. Be firm and insist upon a full explanation. Then, if the hospital tries to give you tests the doctor didn't mention, contact your doctor again and ask what's up.

they should ascertain your problem," she explains.

- Are patients treated in the order of their arrival? Usually not, explains Ms. Thompson. People with the most serious or life-threatening conditions are treated first. Those with the least serious problems are seen last.
- Do hospital personnel ask for your insurance card before taking vital signs or determining what's wrong? That's probably a bad sign. It often means the ER doesn't give priority treatment to those who are badly injured, Ms. Thompson says.

CUTTING COSTS

A long hospital stay can be devastating physically, emotionally and financially. As stratospheric hospital costs leap ever upward, financial trauma is becoming the most frightening aspect of the stay. A couple of weeks in the hospital can wipe out your entire life savings or bury you in debt.

That's why it's important to

COMPARISON SHOPPING

One of the best ways to shave the hospital bill is to practice the same consumer sense you would with any other major purchase. Shop around! Here are some price guidelines based on treatment costs and hospital stay.

- Fractured hip—$4,144 (17 hospital days)
- Having a baby—$2,100 (not

including anesthesia); cesarean section—$3,340
- Hysterectomy—$1,141 (differs greatly by region; New York City—$1,922; Atlanta—$1,078)
- Heart bypass—$15,676
- Heart transplant—$19,118
- Artificial heart—$55,000
- Vasectomy—$241
- Tubal sterilization—$1,180
- Heart attack—$5,300 (10 hospital days)
- Iatrogenic disease (caused by doctor or hospital staff)—$3,517
- Dilation and curettage (D&C)—$1,378 (3.6 hospital days)
- Nose job—$1,399 (3.4 hospital days)
- Broken thighbone—$5,300 (22.7 hospital days)
- Urinalysis—$25 (home tests cost $1)
- Major burn treatment—$26,180
- Surgeons' fees: Appendectomy—$637; hemorrhoidectomy—$405; gallbladder removal—$936; tonsillectomy—$370; radical mastectomy—$1,147
- Per-day hospital room charge—$203 (highest in nation is Washington, D.C.—$285; lowest is South Carolina—$136)

Like a football quarterback on a good day, sometimes saving money at the hospital is all in the timing. To save both time and money, consider that surgical patients can often be admitted to the hospital on the day of the surgery instead of one or two days in advance. All patients should avoid being admitted on Saturday because routine tests and elective surgery will not be done until Monday. The same is true for preholiday admissions. At the other end of a stay, patients should try to be discharged before the weekend.

HEALED IN THE USA

To avoid all the potential problems and worries a hospital can pose, would it be wise for someone seeking good, safe, economical treatment to explore the medical care offered by other countries?

"Probably not," says Stan Foster, M.D., assistant director, International Health, at the U.S. Centers for Disease Control in Atlanta. "U.S. hospitals are equal to or better than those anywhere in the world. There is no reason to travel outside the U.S. A lot of people waste a ton of money searching the world for a cure that doesn't exist."

On the other hand, someone who is not desperately ill might benefit. A study by Steven A. Schroeder, M.D., compared university hospitals in Belgium, West Berlin, the Netherlands and London with his hospital at the University of California, San Francisco (UCSF). He concluded that European university hospitals are larger, less expensive, less technology-intensive, staffed by fewer doctors and occupied by less severely ill patients. The physician rate and cost differences were substantial. In fact, a stay at UCSF can cost up to four times more.

What can you conclude from the study? If you have a major illness that requires advanced technology, or if you require plenty of attention and pampering, you're better off in America. If you have a minor illness—and a strong sense of adventure along with a high tolerance for change, unfamiliar surroundings and doctors who may not speak English—you can save enough cash overseas to combine hospitalization with a European adventure. Call your doctor to see if that's okay—and your travel agent, too, of course.

TIPS FROM X-RAYMAN

Race track regulars know the value of racing forms and tout sheets when it comes time to plunk down their hard-earned cash on a 10- to-1 shot. Racing programs even print the predictions of house handicappers (generally known as Railbird, Trackman and Chartman) to help gamblers win, place or show.

In a more important area, hospital patients are generally given nothing to help them get the most from their stay. Here are some hospital handicapping hints, along with facts and figures from a successful hospital tipster—X-rayman.

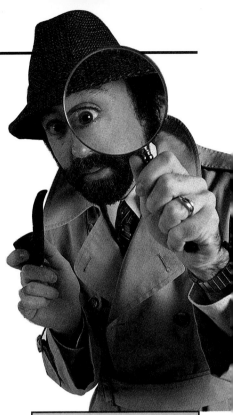

Bill of Wrongs

It's time to see the error of their ways. A survey conducted by a risk-management firm that audits bills exceeding a preset dollar amount has found that a whopping 97.2 percent were inaccurate. Scrutinize those bills!

Avoid Hospitals in July. That's when the new class of residents eagerly emerges from medical school. Up to 85 percent of surgery performed in teaching hospitals is done by residents, so you may end up being some wet-behind-the-scalpel kid's first patient.

Realize That Bigger Isn't Necessarily Better. University of Chicago sociologists surveying hospital patients discovered that those admitted to smaller hospitals were the most satisfied with their care. The hectic, impersonal nature of large hospitals was the key.

Ask about Your Diagnosis. In one study, British researchers discovered that 83 percent of patients they polled favored knowing their disease, 13 percent were indifferent and only 4 percent wanted to be kept in the dark.

Insist on Quiet. Margaret Topf, Ph.D., of the University of California School of Nursing, found that the noise level in the Los Angeles Veterans' Administration Hospital far exceeded the guidelines of 45 decibels set by the Environmental Protection Agency. Dr. Topf found that the hospital averaged 54 decibels, while some rooms had up to 79, the level of a running vacuum cleaner. She suggests hospitals make efforts to still the clatter of equipment. You suggest it, too.

Reserve a Hotel Room. Another study in the "peace and quiet" area determined that hospital patients are subjected to an average of 56 visits a day by doctors, nurses, hospital staff, friends and relatives. The researchers concluded people who need rest are better off in a hotel.

And that's just what some hospitals are doing. Presbyterian-University of Pennsylvania Medical Center in Philadelphia has opened a hotel service for patients recovering from surgery who don't need constant care. The difference in cost is $60 a night compared to $470.

Ask for a Room with a View. Roger S. Ulrich, Ph.D., a geography professor at the University of Delaware, determined that surgery patients with window views of natural settings had shorter stays, complained less and took fewer painkillers than similar patients in identical rooms with no view.

Be an Outpatient. In one survey 75 percent of hospital administrators said their institution will be providing more outpatient care in the coming years. The fastest-growing area is home health care.

Getting Help

Additional sources of hospital help:

• Emergency first aid pamphlet—American College of Emergency Physicians, Communications Department, McNeil Consumer Products Co., Camp Hill Road, Fort Washington, PA 19034
• Pain clinics—The Commission on Accreditation of Rehabilitation Facilities, 25 North Pantano Road, Tucson, AZ 85715
• Reference book—*Take This Book to the Hospital with You:* People's Medical Society, 14 East Minor Street, Emmaus, PA 18049
• To check out a hospital—consult the Joint Commission on Accreditation of Hospitals, 875 North Michigan Avenue, Chicago, IL 60611

Bill of Rights

for Patients

The American Hospital Association has developed a Patients' Bill of Rights to bring about more responsible patient treatment. Here is an adapted version.

1. The patient has the right to considerate and respectful care.

2. The patient has the right to obtain from the physician complete information concerning his or her diagnosis, treatment and prognosis in words the patient can understand.

3. The patient has the right to all information necessary to give informed consent prior to the start of any procedure. This includes the specific procedure or treatment, the risks involved, the duration of incapacitation and possible alternatives.

4. The patient has the right to refuse treatment to the extent permitted by law and to be informed of the medical consequences of his or her action.

5. The patient has the right to privacy concerning his or her medical care. Case discussion, consultation, examination and treatment are confidential.

6. The patient has the right to expect all communications and records to be kept confidential.

7. The patient has the right to expect reasonable response to requests for services. The patient may be transferred to another facility only after receiving complete information on the need for and alternatives to such a transfer.

8. The patient has the right to obtain information as to the relationship of the hospital with various educational and health-care institutions. The patient also has the right to information regarding professional relationships among all those providing treatment.

9. The patient has the right to be informed of experimentation affecting his or her care, and has the right to refuse to participate in such experiments.

10. The patient has the right to continuity of care, including being informed of his or her continuing health care requirements following discharge.

11. The patient has the right to examine and receive an explanation of the bill, regardless of source of payment.

12. The patient has the right to know what hospital rules and regulations apply to his or her conduct as a patient.

For more information on patient rights, consult *The Rights of the Critically Ill* and *The Rights of Doctors and Nurses and Allied Health Professionals*, both from the American Civil Liberties Union, 132 West 43rd Street, New York, NY 10036.

9

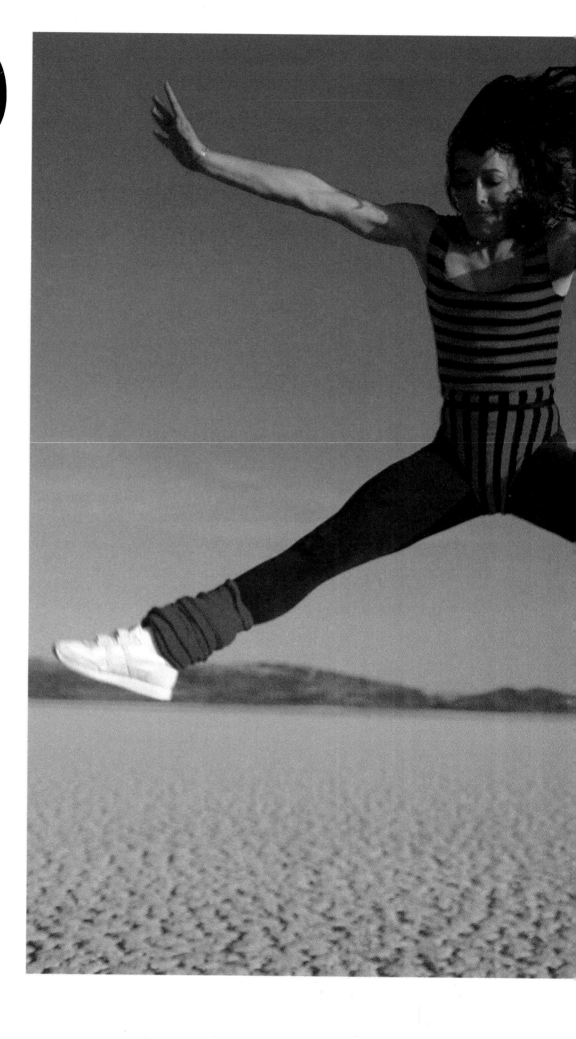

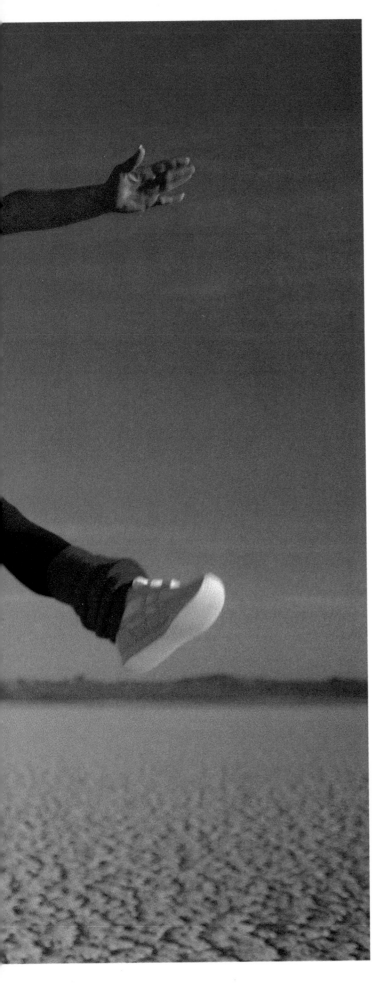

Scoring Your Health Progress

Make today the first day of a healthier life. Use the worksheets to chart your progress.

Strong and lean. Brimming with energy and ready to tackle almost anything, anytime. That's the person most of us would *like* to be, but few of us actually are.

Yet, looking (or at least feeling) like the woman at left is not a hopeless dream. Rather, it's quite an admirable goal, and one you can reach!

What you need to get there is a plan—a *Master* Plan—that incorporates the information you need to improve your health and life. As previous chapters have suggested, the plan focuses on those elements of your lifestyle that are flexible and can provide significant benefits. These elements include your diet, your exercise patterns and your ability to cope with stress.

Maybe such a plan seems *too* simple. It's easier to believe you'd get results from the Fountain of Youth or a year at a Swiss rejuvenation clinic. How can something as simple as walking, say, result in any kind of dramatic improvement? While it's true that occasional walking won't do you a whole lot of good, sticking to a real walking program will strengthen your heart and lungs, make you stronger and maybe even slimmer.

Use the table on page 107 to jot down where you are today. You'll list your weight, blood pressure, blood fat levels and so forth. Using reasonable deadlines, put the plan into action. The next time you hear your friends talking about someone full of pep and vinegar, you might discover they're talking about *you!*

IT'S NEVER TOO LATE TO LEAD A HEALTHY LIFE

Sometimes athletes watch videotapes of themselves in action while their coaches explain how they could have performed better. Improving sports skills is much like improving your health skills: No matter how earnestly you want to improve, you have to recognize your weaknesses and know how to correct your mistakes. And only you can decide which area of health you feel needs the most improvement.

Should you revamp your diet? Experts tell us that the typical diet is too high in cholesterol and saturated fat, sugar, salt, protein and calories and too low in fiber and calcium. Upgrading your diet can be easy. Supermarkets, farmers' markets and corner grocery stores are all chock full of fresh, flavorful foods. Thanks to transportation and refrigeration, the snap beans still have their snap and the cauliflower is snowy white. Oat bran cereal sits near the Wheaties, lean beef and low-salt ham wait in the meat case, and fish—some your mother probably never heard of—rest on their beds of shaved ice. Changing your diet should be, well, a piece of cake.

Yet it often turns out to be one of the most difficult steps in a health-improvement program. Our food choices are strongly influenced by the people with whom we dine, how much time we have to prepare meals, where we find ourselves at mealtime and how much money we have to spend, to name just a few factors. To help you make the right food choices, keep the health benefits foremost in your mind. For example, say you want a double cheeseburger and french fries for lunch. As you push yourself toward the salad bar instead, think about how pleased you'll be when the doctor announces your cholesterol levels have dropped a few points. And your weight has dropped. And you *feel* better. Keep these benefits at the center of your thoughts as you read a menu.

Don't worry if you occasionally treat yourself to ice cream, bacon and eggs or another favorite dish. The important thing is that over the course of time—say, a month—your records show that you are eating more and more first-class foods.

Few jobs demand enough cardiovascular exertion to keep you fit. So if you want to achieve optimal health, you'll probably have to schedule some time for fun and recreation. In return for your hours of exercise you gain flexibility, endurance, strength, agility, relaxation, variety—and an opportunity to either be alone with your thoughts or to socialize with your companions.

Compared with changing your diet, jumping into an exercise program with too much zeal can cause problems. Too much exercise too soon can leave you overtired, sore or injured. So begin slowly. For the first few days be satisfied with the sheer joy of being up and out, taking pride in knowing you've begun a new way of life.

The first few months of your exercise program should focus on building endurance (by means of walking or other aerobic activities) and flexibility (with stretching, for example). Later, work on building strength and coordination. Record the type of activity, duration and distance covered in a pocket diary, chart or log book. (Examples appear in this chapter.) These notes will provide a concrete record of your progress and motivate you to stick with your fitness program.

If you've never worked out before, reaching optimal fitness will probably take 12 to 18 months of conditioning. If you're in moderately good shape, you can expect results in about 6 months. In any case, don't try to increase your activity too quickly. Your body needs about two or three weeks to adapt to one level of fitness before stepping up the pace or workload.

Perhaps the easiest part of your health lifestyle to improve is stress management. Choose the method that suits you best—imagery, Progressive Relaxation or deep breathing, to name a few. You can start immediately—and feel the benefits after just one session.

Improving your personal health scoreboard doesn't have to take hours a day. Thirty minutes a day spent exercising, planning healthier meals or practicing a relaxation technique is an investment of just 2 percent of your daily time—an investment in improving your quality of life and increasing the odds of it being a long and healthy one.

Where You Are

Weight	
Blood pressure	
Heart rate (resting)	
Cholesterol level HDL level (ratio)	
Triglyceride level	
Number of X-rays	
Vision	
Hearing	
Number of visits to dentist per year	

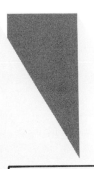

Number of visits to doctor in last year	For inoculation	
	For illness	
	For accident	
	Other	
Exercise (hours per week)		
Practice Stress Management		

Changes You Can Make

Goal	Reasonable Deadline
Stop smoking	1 week
Lose weight	1 to 1½ lb. per week
Exercise 3 times per week	Today
Lower blood pressure	2 to 3 months
Reduce cholesterol to 220 mg. or less	3 months
Practice stress coping	Today

Your body will begin to grow stronger and healthier the moment you take your first positive steps toward optimal health. This chart shows which areas you can control and how soon you can expect to achieve your goals.

Menu Planning

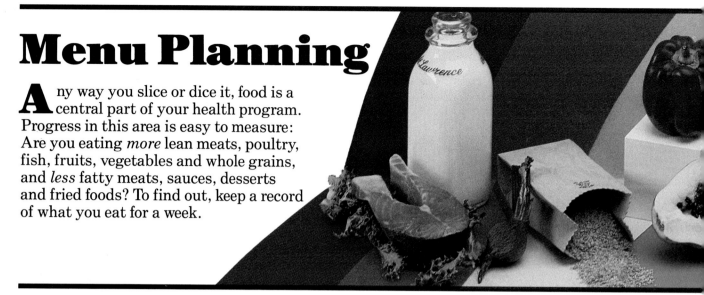

Any way you slice or dice it, food is a central part of your health program. Progress in this area is easy to measure: Are you eating *more* lean meats, poultry, fish, fruits, vegetables and whole grains, and *less* fatty meats, sauces, desserts and fried foods? To find out, keep a record of what you eat for a week.

Meat, Poultry and Fish

1. Choose red meats carefully. The best are leaner cuts with as much fat removed as possible. Meat that is processed into links, cold cuts or patties often contains too much fat, as well as additives—used mostly to add shelf life and color—that have been linked to cancer.

2. Replace some of the meat on your menu with poultry and fowl: chicken, turkey, pheasant, quail and so forth. They're packed with iron, zinc, niacin and vitamin B$_6$. Remove the skin from poultry to cut fat content. When considering poultry as an alternative to red meat, don't forget to count meals you eat away from home.

3. Fish has less saturated fat and calories than the leanest meat or poultry. In fact, you can eat fish without a trace of guilt. So give this solid source of protein a leading role on your menu. Tuna, halibut, cod, flounder, haddock, pollock, mullet, ocean perch, carp, whiting—and seafood such as crab, scallops and lobster—have less than 5 percent fat.

Vegetables

1. Leafy greens are good as gold. So load up on Swiss chard, spinach, cabbage, kale, brussels sprouts and collards every chance you get. They're good sources of vitamins A and C and B vitamins and supply some potassium, magnesium and iron. And they're deliciously low in calories.

2. Don't forget to include the plain but nourishing roots and tubers. Potatoes, for example, are a good source of fiber, vitamin C, certain B vitamins and minerals. Garlic and onions contain natural components that seem to exert a protective effect against heart disease. Carrots and sweet potatoes are high in beta-carotene, which may help to prevent cancer.

3. Raw or cooked, the stem and flower vegetables such as broccoli and asparagus are crunchy ways to get vitamins A and C, minerals and other nutrients. Let flowering vegetables such as peppers, eggplant, tomatoes, pumpkins and squash fill out your menu. Ounce for ounce, peppers surpass oranges as a source of vitamin C.

Fruits

1. Don't think of oranges and grapefruits as breakfast foods only. Citrus fruits make great midday or midnight snacks. And lemonade is an excellent, C-rich alternative to soft drinks when you need to quench your thirst.

2. Take a pear to lunch. Bring home a peach. Make life a bowl of cherries. Fresh fruits with seeds or stones are generally high in vitamin A, low in calories and about as succulent a sandwich mate as you're likely to find anywhere.

3. How nutritious can a little berry be? Very. One-half cup of strawberries, for example, packs about two-thirds the RDA of vitamin C for an adult. Other berries aren't pikers, though: All contain fair amounts of vitamin C, some fiber—and few calories. Try blackberries, loganberries, mulberries, raspberries, blueberries and cranberries. They're all berry good.

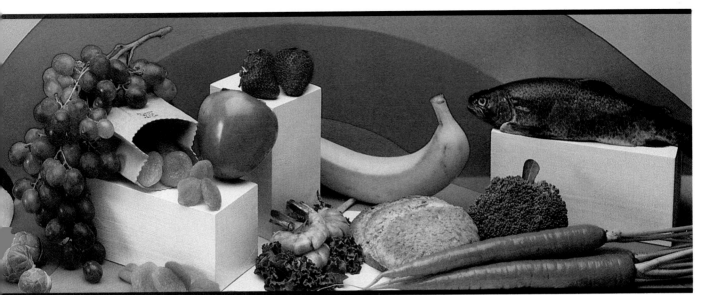

4. Low-fat cooking methods such as broiling, poaching, steaming and baking are better methods for preparing meat, poultry, fish and game than frying. After all, what's the sense of replacing the fat you avoided at the store with fat you add at the stove?

Food	Times per Week

4. Beans and peas supply a fair share of calcium and certain B vitamins. But they're best known for a nutrient other vegetables lack almost totally: protein, which they supply without the fat that usually accompanies animal protein. Choose from kidney, pinto, Great Northern, yellow, green or lima beans, sweet peas or snow peas.

Food	Times per Week

4. Think "globes" for vitamins C and A. Like many orange-colored fruits and vegetables, cantaloupes are rich in beta-carotene, the precursor of vitamin A. Honeydews and cantaloupes are both rich in vitamin C and minerals such as potassium and calcium. And they're *so* refreshing!

Food	Times per Week

Grains, Breads and Cereals

1. Whole wheat and other whole grain breads are wonderful sources of many of the B vitamins, especially thiamine and riboflavin (B_1 and B_2). By switching from white to whole wheat, you'll also get more minerals, such as potassium, magnesium and zinc.

2. Brown rice has three times more fiber than unenriched white rice, almost five times more thiamine, three times more niacin, three times more B_6, twice as much iron, three times more magnesium, five times more vitamin E and 50 percent more zinc. That's enough of a difference to warrant frequent appearances of brown rice on the dinner table.

3. Oat bran may help lower cholesterol levels in the blood. That's probably enough reason to eat it, but luckily it's also delicious. Make room for oat bran muffins and rolled oats on your breakfast menu.

Nuts and Seeds

1. Raw, unsalted almonds and peanuts, like all nuts, are relatively high in calories. But they supply respectable amounts of protein, B vitamins, vitamin E and magnesium. Almonds also supply fair amounts of calcium. Unroasted almonds and peanuts, then, make better snacks than potato chips or pretzels.

2. Walnuts, filberts, pistachios and Brazil nuts supply varying amounts of potassium, iron and thiamine. But buy them only for Thanksgiving. They have some redeeming value as an occasional treat, but they're high in fat.

3. Sesame seeds, pumpkin seeds and sunflower seeds are leading sources of protein, fiber, B vitamins, calcium, potassium, iron and zinc. Ounce for ounce, pumpkin seeds pack nearly as much protein as porterhouse steak. And they're one of the richest sources of zinc you can find. So seeds get high marks, but only if you are not watching your weight.

Milk Products and Eggs

1. Best bets from the dairy case are skim milk, plain low-fat yogurt, low-fat cottage cheese and part-skim mozzarella. Nonfat dry milk and evaporated milk are also excellent. They supply protein, calcium and the B vitamin riboflavin, but do not contain large amounts of fat.

2. Cheese is a concentrated form of milk—and all of milk's components, good or bad. So while cheddar and many other popular cheeses are good sources of calcium and protein, they also can be filled with fat. Eat them only occasionally and in moderation. Those on a salt-restricted diet may have to avoid cheese entirely.

3. If it weren't for cholesterol, eggs would be the perfect food. They offer lots of protein and a smattering of nearly all other nutrients. But because cholesterol has been linked to heart disease, people with heart disease should avoid them. Everyone else can probably eat eggs once or twice a week with no problem.

Candy, Pastry and Sweets

1. If you're trying to lose weight without success, perhaps you're eating more high-calorie sweets than you realize. For a week or two, keep a written record of every cookie, cupcake and candy bar you eat. No cheating! Then cut in half the number of servings you eat of these foods every week.

2. If you can afford the calories, you can eat dessert. Just use common sense to make sure those extra calories contain some nutrition. And steer clear of desserts that are high in fat, such as cheesecake.

3. Need a sudden burst of power? If you're already exercising—5 miles into a 10-mile hike, for instance—a handful of raisins or a candy bar can give you the immediate energy you need to keep going.

4. Don't bypass foods made from lesser-known grains such as millet and bulgur. These grains are high in the B vitamin thiamine and in the minerals iron and magnesium. And they're versatile. Cooked bulgur, for example, can be eaten for breakfast as a cereal, used to extend meat dishes or added to soup in the same way as noodles.

Food	Times per Week

4. Save cashews and pecans for your next Halley's Comet party. They're so fatty that you should eat them once in a blue moon. And people with high blood pressure should beware: Salted peanuts may contain up to 82 times the sodium in unsalted peanuts.

Food	Times per Week

4. Ice cream, cream cheese, whipped cream, butter, sour cream and fried eggs are too high in fat and low in other nutrients to show up regularly on your menu. View them as the special treats they really are, and save them for appropriate occasions.

Food	Times per Week

4. If your problem is cavities, not calories, the *kind* of sweets you eat makes a difference. Avoid those gooey sweets such as caramels, jelly beans, toffee and fudge, which tend to cling to your teeth, promoting decay.

Food	Times per Week

Charting Your Exercise Progress

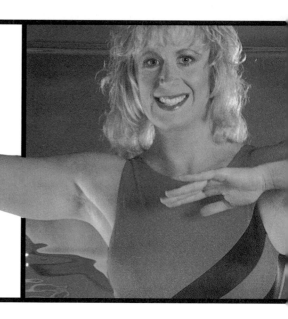

A vigorous jog through the park—or any other activity that gets your heart pumping for 30 minutes or more—can improve your health in dozens of ways. The best exercise program is one that includes activities that build strength, endurance and flexibility. Choose the combination that appeals to *you*.

Strength

1. Nautilus and Universal equipment is found in most gyms and fitness clubs. It builds strength by working each muscle group against weights that you increase as you grow stronger. (And that you can't drop on your toes!) Start with light weights and work up slowly.

2. Free weights—barbells and dumbbells—work much like Nautilus and Universal equipment to build strength and tone the entire body. Their advantages: They're less expensive than more elaborate equipment, should you prefer to work out at home, and they take up less room if you live in small quarters. A disadvantage: They require more skill to use properly.

3. Perform about 12 repetitions at about 50 percent of your maximum lift with each free-weight position or weight machine. That's 1 set. Then move on to the next position or machine. Allow your muscles to rest for 48 hours between strength-training sessions. Or work different muscle groups on alternate days.

Endurance

1. Working out for longer distances, longer times, or both, increases your endurance. Staying power prevents fatigue and injury during long runs, bike races, day-long hikes or other sustained activity.

2. Aerobic exercises such as running, biking, swimming, rope-skipping, rowing and cross-country skiing build endurance by improving the efficiency of your heart and lungs. Work hard enough so that you're slightly out of breath but can still carry on a conversation. Schedule at least 30 minutes of aerobic activity 3 times a week or more.

3. Want to increase strength *and* endurance? Circuit training alternates 30-second bursts of weight lifting with 30 seconds of aerobic exercise. Begin with a set of leg-extension exercises, for example, then jump rope for 30 seconds. Without pausing, work your biceps, then jog in place and so on, for 30 to 45 minutes.

Flexibility

1. The farther you can reach, twist, turn, swing and bend, the more flexible you are. Flexibility keeps you supple, loose and less prone to strain and injury. One way to measure the flexibility of your back is by trying to touch your toes. If you get only as far as your calves, your whole body could probably benefit from some stretching exercises.

2. Gentle stretching can greatly improve your mobility. Start easy, with a daily routine of arm stretches, side stretches, leg stretches and back stretches. Take a deep breath after each stretch. Begin with 1 set of stretches and work up to 2 or 3.

3. One of the best ways to increase your flexibility is with yoga, the Eastern art of toning and stretching the body. And we're not talking superdifficult pretzel poses. Most good books on yoga include an easy-to-follow routine that is so relaxing it will give you both physical *and* mental flexibility.

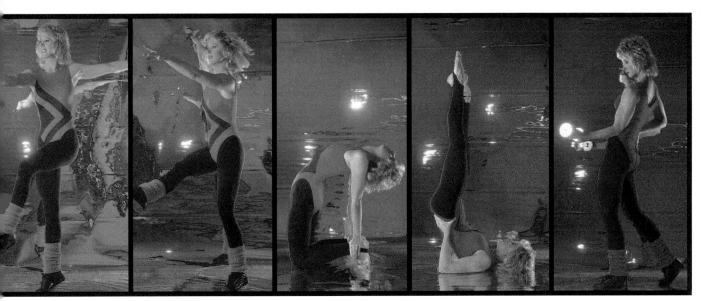

4. If you decide to work out with weights, ask a qualified coach or instructor how to use the equipment correctly. You can't fully benefit from weight training unless you use the equipment properly. And you'll avoid hurting yourself or damaging the equipment.

Strength Training	Times per Week

4. Don't feel obligated to exercise until you drop. If you're tired or sense any muscle fatigue, slow down, even if it means changing your workout schedule. Work hard when you feel strong, but be on the alert for what your body may be telling you. (Everyone, from beginners to seasoned athletes, experiences an occasional off day—or off *week*.)

Endurance (aerobic activity)	Times per Week

4. Practicing good posture, too, can limber you up and relieve stress and strain on your joints, especially if you have to sit or stand for long periods of time. Practice standing erect, with an imaginary vertical line extending from just behind one ear to your ankle. To sit erect, tilt your upper pelvis foward and upward.

Flexibility Activity	Times per Week

Stress Management

Bank overdrafts. Computer snafus. Car trouble. Such minor but frequent troubles are enough to make you cry. Or scream. Or both. To enjoy life, you need to cope with the physical and mental tension called stress. Start by getting your Minimum Daily Requirement of fun, plus a daily dose of R & R. And finish by learning to succeed at the things that count—and not buckle under trivial frustrations.

Fun

1. Play is not optional—it's a must for good health. Why should kids have a monopoly on good times? It doesn't matter how you amuse yourself—playing Scrabble, learning new dance steps, tossing a Frisbee for Fido—as long as you enjoy yourself. Review your daily routine. Do you regularly set aside time for a good time?

2. Learn to laugh at yourself. Nobody's perfect. If you make a mistake, try to see the humor in it. If someone else does something dumb, try to appreciate the humor in the situation. Sometimes a good-natured chuckle can take the edge off a touchy situation—making life easier for all concerned.

3. Be a little bit daring. Try new experiences, new foods, new clothing. Dress up for Halloween. Test-drive a sports car. Tie a balloon to your desk at work. Whatever you do, never say, "I'm too old" or "I'm not the type." Be adventuresome!

Coping Techniques

1. Meditate. Find a quiet place and meditate for 10 minutes twice a day, every day. The easiest method is the Relaxation Response, developed by Herbert Benson, M.D. Relax all of your muscles. Say the word *one* with each slow, deliberate exhalation of breath. When a thought comes, don't resist it—just easily return your attention to the word. And to inner peace.

2. Use Progressive Relaxation. Sit in a comfortable chair. Make a fist with one hand. Hold it for several seconds. Then relax. Note the difference between the feelings of tension and relaxation. Repeat the exercise with each muscle group of your body. Finish by tensing and relaxing your facial muscles. The whole process should take about 20 minutes.

3. Breathe deeply. If you feel overwhelmed by stress—or if you sense a wave of anxiety building inside you—take a deep breath. Hold it for a moment, then exhale slowly. Repeat this process several times. (You may also combine deep breathing with imagery: Imagine yourself in a safe, stress-free situation to rescue yourself from pressure.)

Success

1. Think of success as a *journey,* not a destination. And don't expect instant results. Too often, we equate success with a single goal: graduation, a promotion, buying a dream house. Reaching the goal can, ironically, lead to a big letdown. Ultimate success is really a series of small, difficult steps—and some failures—strung together.

2. Banish negative terms from your vocabulary. Statements prefaced by "I can't"; "I don't"; "I never" can only lead to failure. You're much more likely to reach your goals if you think like a winner. Assume that you have the smarts, aptitude or agility to accomplish new tasks.

3. Negotiate for what you want. Learning how to bargain, compromise and share can get you more out of life: love, money, prestige, security, justice and freedom. In fact, anything worth having often requires the favor and cooperation of others.

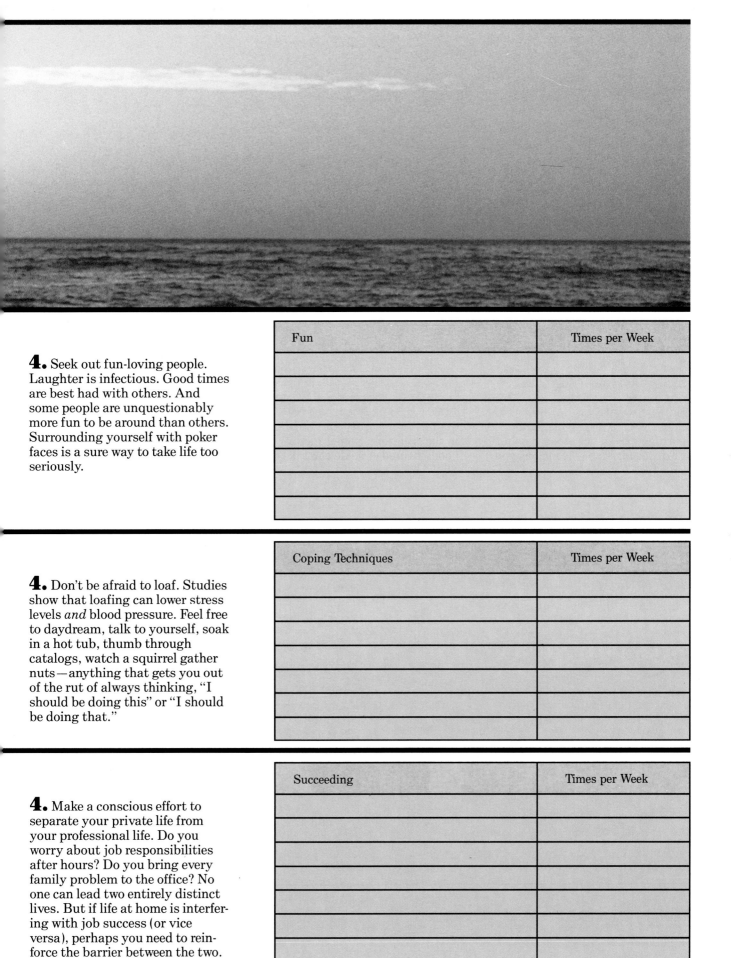

4. Seek out fun-loving people. Laughter is infectious. Good times are best had with others. And some people are unquestionably more fun to be around than others. Surrounding yourself with poker faces is a sure way to take life too seriously.

Fun	Times per Week

4. Don't be afraid to loaf. Studies show that loafing can lower stress levels *and* blood pressure. Feel free to daydream, talk to yourself, soak in a hot tub, thumb through catalogs, watch a squirrel gather nuts—anything that gets you out of the rut of always thinking, "I should be doing this" or "I should be doing that."

Coping Techniques	Times per Week

4. Make a conscious effort to separate your private life from your professional life. Do you worry about job responsibilities after hours? Do you bring every family problem to the office? No one can lead two entirely distinct lives. But if life at home is interfering with job success (or vice versa), perhaps you need to reinforce the barrier between the two.

Succeeding	Times per Week

10

Chill
f

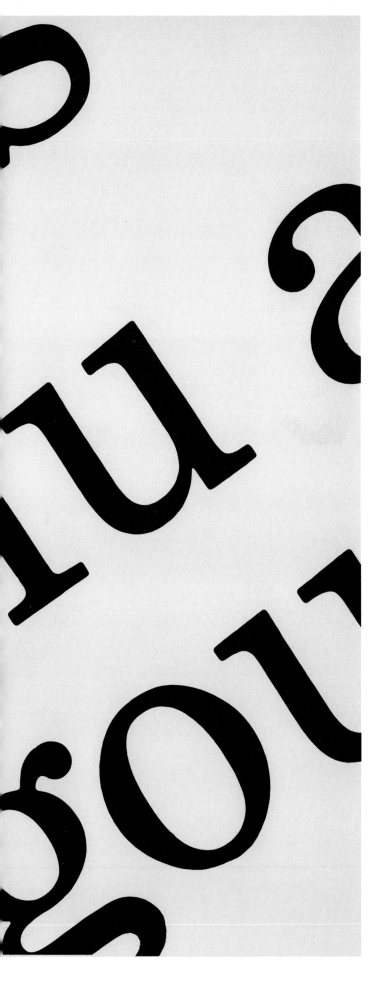

Index of Symptoms and Conditions

No need to pore through each index of The Prevention Total Health System.® Use this handy guide to find common symptoms and health conditions.

Suppose you have a cough and you want to know what's causing it. Should you look up Bronchitis? Allergy? Common cold? Pneumonia? Where do you begin to find the information you need?

You begin, quite simply, by looking under the heading "Cough." Our master index of symptoms and conditions has done the work for you, listing symptoms discussed in the Prevention Total Health System® books. The listings are in alphabetical order. And each listing will tell you where to find the information you seek in any of the books that has discussed it.

Suppose, for example, you look up the listing for cough. What would you find? The references use the initials of the book's title, followed by a page number. (See the key on the first page of the index.) One listing for cough, for example, might be "UMW28-29." It sends you to the volume *Using Medicines Wisely* (UMW), where you will learn on page 29 that if your cough is "productive" you should avoid using medicines that act as cough suppressants. The index also will refer you to EHH (*Everyday Health Hints*) page 47, where you will discover the seven signs that tell you when a cough means real trouble. And in EH (*Emotional Health*) on page 51 you'll discover what effects cough medicines can have upon your mental health.

If you prefer to look up a health condition, that's easily done, too, as they are listed here. Also, at the end of this volume there is a complete index of every topic discussed in The Prevention Total Health System.®

A

The Prevention Total Health System® Multi-Volume Index

Source Notes

Chapter 1

Page 2

"The Doctor Glut" adapted from "Is the Doctor Surplus for Real?" by Merian Kirchner, *Medical Economics*, October, 1983.

Chapter 2

Page 17

"Erin Go Broccoli!" adapted from "Diet and 20-Year Mortality from Coronary Heart Disease: The Ireland-Boston Diet-Heart Study" by Lawrence H. Kushi, S.C.D., et al., *New England Journal of Medicine*, March 28, 1985. Reprinted by permission of the publisher.

Page 18

"Food Sources of Key Nutrients" adapted from *Composition of Foods: Vegetables and Vegetable Products*, Agricultural Handbook No. 8-11, by Nutrition Monitoring Division (Washington, D.C.: Human Nutrition Information Service, U.S. Department of Agriculture, 1984) and *Composition of Foods: Fruits and Fruit Juices*, Agricultural Handbook No. 8-9, by Consumer Nutrition Center (Washington, D.C.: U.S. Department of Agriculture, 1982) and *Composition of Foods: Dairy and Egg Products*, Agricultural Handbook No. 8-1, by Consumer and Food Economics Institute (Washington, D.C.: Agricultural Research Service, U.S. Department of Agriculture, 1976) and *Nutritive Value of American Foods in Common Units*, Agriculture Handbook No. 456, by Catherine F. Adams (Washington, D.C.: Agricultural Research Service, U.S. Department of Agriculture, 1975) and *Pantothenic Acid, Vitamin B_6 and Vitamin B_{12},* Home Economics Research Report No. 36, by Martha Louise Orr (Wash-ington, D.C.: Agricultural Research Service, U.S. Department of Agriculture, 1969) and "Folacin in Selected Foods," by Betty P. Perloff and R. R. Butrum, *Journal of the American Dietetic Association*, February, 1977 and *Composition of Foods: Poultry Products*, Agriculture Handbook No. 8-5, by Consumer and Food Economics Institute (Washington, D.C.: Science and Education Administration, U.S. Department of Agriculture, 1979) and "Zinc Content of Selected Foods," by Jeanne H. Freeland and Robert Cousins, *Journal of the American Dietetic Association*, June, 1976 and "Provisional Tables on the Zinc Content of Foods," by Elizabeth W. Murphy, Barbara Wells Willis and Bernice K. Watt, *Journal of the American Dietetic Association*, April, 1975.

Pages 20-21

"The Master Target" prepared in cooperation with Annette B. Natow, Ph.D., R.D., and Jo-Ann Heslin, M.A., R.D.

Chapter 3

Page 36

"Weekend Fitness" prepared by Bryant Stamford, Ph.D., Exercise Physiology Laboratory, University of Louisville School of Medicine, Louisville, Ky.

Chapter 4

Page 49

"Henny Youngman's Best One-Liners" reprinted by permission of the author from *Take My Jokes, Please*, by Henny Youngman (New York: Richardson & Snyder, 1983).

Chapter 5

Page 58

"Indoor Air Pollution" table courtesy of the Bonneville Power Administration, Portland, Oregon.

Compiled with additional information from the U.S. Environmental Protection Agency and the U.S. Consumer Product Safety Commission and "Possible Carcinogenic Components of Indoor Air-Combustion By-products, Formaldehyde, Mineral Fibers, Radiation, and Tobacco Smoke," by T. D. Sterling and A. Arundel, *Journal of Environmental Science and Health*, vol. C2, no. 2, 1984 and "An Overview of Indoor Air Quality," by Jerome J. Wesolowski, *Journal of Environmental Health*, May/June, 1984 and "Radon and Its Progeny in the Indoor Environment," by Mark Tartaglia, Salvatore R. DiNardi and Jerry Ludwig, *Journal of Environmental Health*, September/October, 1984 and "Indoor Air Pollution: A Public Health Perspective," by John D. Spengler and Ken Sexton, *Science*, July, 1983 and *Air-to-Air Heat Exchangers for Houses*, by William A. Shureliff (Andover, Mass.: Brick House Publishing, 1982).

Page 60

"Cigarettes—The Ingredients Label Would Read . . ." compiled from information provided by Department of National Health and Welfare, Canada; The American Conference of Governmental Hygienists, Inc.; The International Agency for Research on Cancer; and the U.S. Department of Health and Human Services.

Chapter 7

Pages 81-89

Information in this chapter is adapted from *How to Choose a Good Doctor*, by George D. LeMaitre, M.D., F.A.C.S. (Andover, Mass.: Andover Publishing Group, 1979).

Page 83

"Your Doctor's Report Card" adapted from "Peo-ple's Medical Society Physician Evaluation Form," from the People's Medical Society, Emmaus, Pa.

Page 84

"Who's Who" adapted from *Getting the Most Out of Your Doctor*, by Lawrence A. May, M.D. (New York: Basic Books, 1977).

Chapter 8

Page 105

"Bill of Rights for Patients" adapted by permission of the publisher from "A Patient's Bill of Rights," by the American Hospital Association (Chicago: American Hospital Association, 1975).

Chapter 9

Page 107

"Where You Are/Where You Want to Be" compiled from information provided by Isadore Rosenfeld, M.D., New York, N.Y.

Photography Credits

Cover: Mark Bricklin: top left. Angelo Caggiano: center right. Carl Doney: bottom right. Mitchell T. Mandell: top right. Paul Pelak: bottom left. Margaret Skrovanek: center left.
Staff Photographers— Angelo Caggiano: pp. viii-1; 28-29; 66-67; 90-91. Carl Doney: pp. 26-27; 33; 46; 52-53; 65, top right; 75, top. T. L. Gettings: pp. 114-115. John P. Hamel: p. 65, bottom. Donna Hornberger: pp. 9; 63; 69; 70-71; 75, bottom; 80-81. Mitchell T. Mandell: pp. 108-109. Alison Miksch: pp. 12-13; 22-23; 24; 77. Margaret Skrovanek: pp. 47; 64, bottom. Sally Shenk Ullman: p. 101.

Other Photographers— Julian Baum: pp. 34; 104-105. Paul Boyer: p. 35. Michael Kevin Daly: pp. 42-43. Roy Gumple: p. 32. Don Hamerman: p. 40. Leo de Wys, Inc.: p. 64, top left; Seymour

Linden: p. 64, top right.
David Madison: p. 39.
Paul Pelak: pp. 112-113.
Sue Tom: p. 41, bottom.

Additional Photographs Courtesy of—Photo Researchers, Inc.: p. 65, top left. Dorothy Saling: p. 41, top. Star File Photos: p. 11, inset. Wide World Photos, Inc.: p. 11, top.

Photographic Styling Credits—Barbara Fritz: p. 24. Kay Seng Lichthardt: p. 46. Debra Minotti: pp. 66-67; 90-91.

Illustration Credits
Bascove: pp. 36; 38; 79; 99; 100. Susan Blubaugh: pp. 18, 50-51. Mellisa Edmonds: pp. 2; 17; 21; 82-83. Lynn Foulk: p. 15. Susan Gray: pp. 55; 56; 57; 93. Mary Anne Shea: pp. 13-14; 24-25; 59; 98. Elwood Smith: pp. 19; 86-87; 96. Wendy Wray: p. 68.

Index

Rodale Press, Inc., publishes PREVENTION®, the better health magazine.
For information on how to order your subscription,
write to PREVENTION®, Emmaus, PA 18049.